BROKEN

How the broken mental health care system leads to broken lives and broken hearts.

by Linda Comac

ISBN 978-1-706-95907-6

Dedication

To Erik and Ainsley Jacobs,
whose love and support keep the broken pieces from flying apart.

To Tema Goetzel,
the big sister who has always held my hand.

To Ilene Johnson and Warren Goetzel,
for their unbroken love.

And it has come to pass
a path set in stone now breaks like glass.
The failings of yesterday become my catalyst,
I seek the guidance gained from silence.
Illumination from within the darkness.
My council kept with the emptiness,
in the heart of the unknown.

By Alan Jacobs

Table of Contents

Prologue

My beloved son Alan lost his battle with depression, anxiety, and chronic pain on January 10, 2015, when, two weeks before his 29th birthday, he died of an accidental prescription drug overdose.

This bright, witty, loving young man had been plagued by anxiety, back pain, and depression, exacerbated by a too-sensitive nature: any pain he saw, he felt; any injustice he recognized, he wanted to correct. Although Alan could not find a way to fight the demons that beset him, he was always ready to defend those who were doing battle with problems or foes: he was just as quick with an assertive stance as he was with sage advice.

Tragically, there were few sages among the many mental health professionals he had consulted over the years. Not one of them even considered that he might be suffering from post-traumatic stress disorder (PTSD). Instead, they treated him for ADHD — with pills; later, for childhood depression — with pills; still later for anxiety and back pain — with pills.

Towards the end of his life, Alan experienced two non-lethal overdoses but he continued to take the drugs that were prescribed for him. After all, physicians, the media and pharmaceutical companies had trained him to believe in the power of the pill.

If psychological pain and anxiety motivated Alan's final act, what motivated the pain and anxiety that led him to drugs in the first place? Why did more than 20 years of testing and of meeting with psychologists, psychiatrists, social workers and special education teachers never get to the root of the problem? If he lived with depression, anxiety, and pain throughout his life, why did no intervention stop him from arriving at his final moment? Why? Because the mental health system is broken and people — especially mothers — are imperfect. There's more than enough blame to go around...

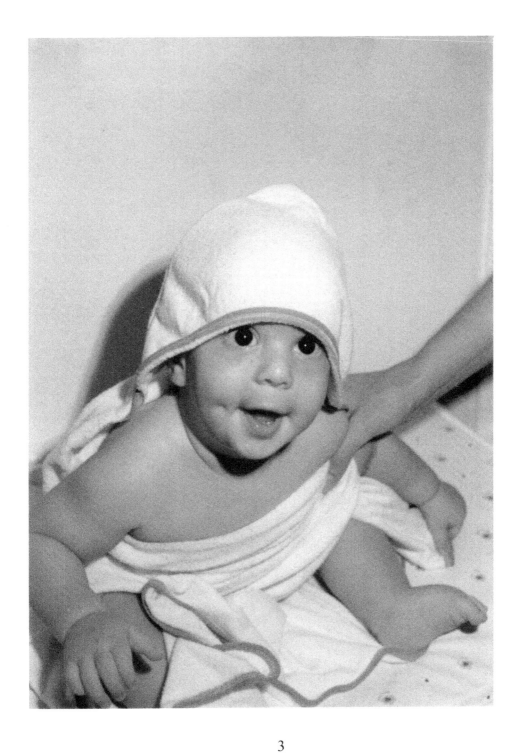

3

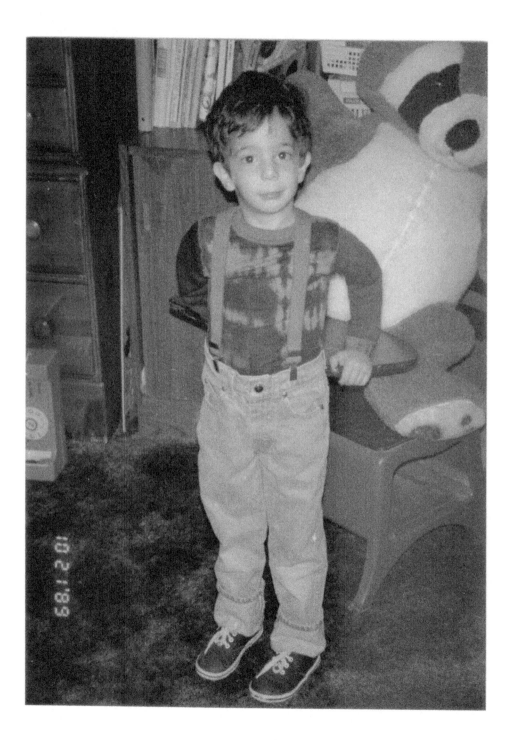

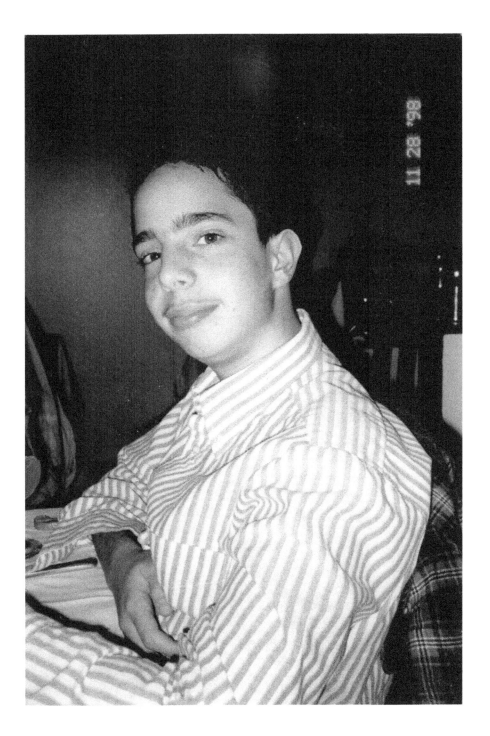

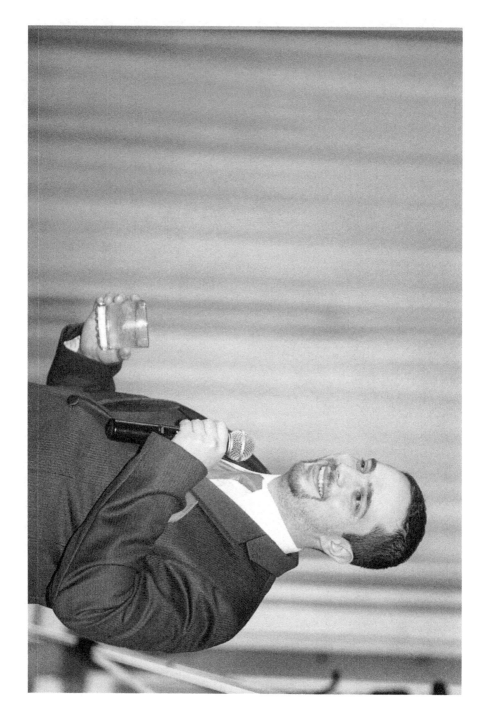

Introduction

I am a vessel.
I am a vessel without destination, devoid of direction.
No roles define me, yet conflict embraces me.
At the mercy of lucidity,
I am adrift in a world all too real.
A hollow man.
Into the arms of eternal struggle,
I must condemn my restless mind.
And it has come to pass,
a path set in stone now breaks like glass.
The failings of yesterday become
the catalyst to seek my change.
And it has come to pass,
a path set in stone now breaks like glass.
The failings of yesterday become my catalyst,
I seek the guidance gained from silence.
Illumination from within the darkness.
My council kept with the emptiness,
in the heart of the unknown.

by Alan Jacobs

"Mentally ill" — the term conjures up images of crazed shooters, wild-eyed people who push others off subway platforms, and unkempt cackling hags who forage for food in garbage cans. The facts paint a different picture.

Studies show that the vast majority of those who commit violent acts do not have a mental illness.[1] In reality, those who have severe mental illness are ten times more likely to be attacked, raped, or mugged than those in the general population.[2]

More than two-thirds of the 11.4 million Americans who have a mental illness lead productive lives right beside us in our communities. Yet fear and stigma concerning mental illness persist — sometimes with tragic consequences. Many who might otherwise seek treatment do not do so because they are afraid of being ridiculed and shunned. It has been reported that "up to 75 percent of Americans and Europeans don't seek the help they need."[3]

Mental illnesses are more common than cancer, diabetes or heart disease: about one in four people over the age of 18 has a diagnosable mental disorder.[4] These people can recover or manage their illnesses and lead happy, healthy, productive lives.[5] In order to do so, they need rehabilitation, talk therapy, self-help skills, and — in some circumstances — even medication or a combination of these. Most importantly, they need the acceptance, support, and understanding of family and friends.

The fear of being shunned, treated like lepers of old, or whispered about behind closed doors prevents many from even seeking the treatment they need. According to the World Health Organization (WHO) nearly two-thirds of people with a known mental disorder never seek help from a health professional. Stigma, discrimination, and neglect prevent care and treatment from reaching people with mental disorders.[6]

The public's misunderstanding of mental illness doesn't help. People aren't even aware of how common mental health problems are until there are celebrity suicides or when police intervention in a mental health crisis is required. We cry for celebrities like Robin Williams and Phillip Seymour Hoffman who take their own lives, romanticizing them as artists with tortured souls. We are shocked by the headlines about the use of police force to control a mentally ill person. Those who bear their burdens day in and day out without making headlines are simply ignored.

Sadly, a good number of those who do seek treatment cannot find the help they need; mental health resources are sorely lacking. According to the U.S. Office of Adolescent Health, "…mental health care is frequently difficult to access. In 2013, 10 percent of adolescents lacked insurance; even when they are covered, the amount of mental health services they can receive is often limited."[7]

The numbers speak volumes: In 2017, only 42.6 percent of the 46.6 million adults with a mental illness had received mental health services in the past year.[8] At that time, there were 37,679 state psychiatric beds, down 13 percent from 2010.[9] A 2018 report indicated that, on average, there are only 9.35 psychiatrists per 100,000 people. Almost 4,000 areas in the U.S. have shortages of mental health care professionals. More than 50% of the country lacks sufficient practitioners to meet the needs of their area.[10]

Such woefully inadequate resources constitute a crisis in an era when mental health services are so desperately needed. Neuropsychiatric disorders are the leading cause of disability in the U.S.[11] Life expectancy in 2017 fell to an average of 78.6 years for the total U.S. population, down from 78.7 years in 2016, due largely to the rise in drug overdoses and suicide.[12] "Suicide is increasing against the backdrop of generally declining mortality, and is currently one of the 10 leading causes of death overall and within each age group 10–64."[13]

This myriad of sources begins to paint a picture showing that the mental health system in the U.S. is broken and desperately needs to be repaired. If the system is not repaired, large numbers of people with mental health problems may not seek help, may not be able to find help, or may not be adequately treated when they do find help. Families will be broken by fear, frustration, and – all too often – loss. I know. I've walked both paths — as the parent of a child with a mental illness and as a person diagnosed with a mental illness.

You may question how important it is to you personally whether good mental health care is readily available. After all, there are so many other chronic, debilitating, and fatal diseases that require attention. Cancer, heart disease, diabetes, Alzheimer's, and other maladies rob people of their lives and dramatically affect friends, family, and finances.

The effects of mental illness on a family are also dramatic. In a home where someone is afflicted by mental illness, family life is often so unpredictable that it becomes impossible to plan for something as simple as nightly dinners.

As with any chronic disease, the demands of the mentally ill person can intrude into and even take over the lives of those around them. Siblings of the ill person may feel ignored and resentful. The relationship between parents can become strained as they often argue about the best course of action and where or whether blame should be assigned. Feelings of anger, resentment, and guilt slowly eat away at the fabric of a family. The emotional and behavioral consequences for everyone can include insomnia, migraines, anxiety, depression, and social withdrawal.

It's no wonder that the National Institute of Mental Health calculates that mental illness accounts for more than 15 percent of the burden of disease in the USA — more than the disease burden caused by cardiovascular and circulatory diseases combined.[14] It also far surpasses the disease burden brought about by violence or transportation accidents.[14] Major depressive disorder is the leading cause of disability for those between the ages of 15 and 44.[15] These statistics will not improve until or unless those suffering from mental illness can overcome the hurdles they face and ultimately get the help they so desperately need.

This book begins with the story of my younger son's lifelong battle with depression and anxiety — two disorders that fall under the heading of "mental illness." It is also tells the story of my own encounters with the mental health system when I was diagnosed with "acute geriatric depression."

These stories of real life suffering are considered anecdotal evidence. Generally speaking, the scientific community shuns such evidence.

However, there are many stories like mine. Given enough anecdotes, a clear trend emerges. Sadly, my son's story, as well as my own, fit all too well inside the picture painted by the studies and organizations.

Much needs to be done to ensure that all Americans can live fully functioning lives of dignity and worth. To start, we must remove the stigma and fear and replace it with understanding —understanding not only of those who suffer from mental illness, but of the problems that beset the mental health system.

PART ONE

Tread purposefully
we of no consequence
for no heart beats for you
save your own
Tread softly
we of deep breath and sigh
for why conspire
when truth stands alone
Tread eternally
we of tortured soul
for the path ahead
is an ever winding road

Wanderer, by Alan Jacobs

A Broken Life

Every child arrives in the world as a blank canvas. The borders of the painting may well be determined by nature, but life's experiences fill the spaces in between. For some, the canvas will someday be awash in the warm hues of sunshine while, for others, darkness and shadow will come to predominate.

It often feels that, from the very first moments, the brush painting the canvas of Alan Ross Jacobs's life was held by a less-than benevolent Fate. Looking back, it seems that from the moment of his conception, fate was loading his palette with the darkest of colors.

At a glance, Alan's canvas seemed as if it should have been boundless. His parents and grandparents were highly intelligent and well-educated—three of his four grandparents were college graduates in an era when such a feat was far from commonplace. Both of Alan's paternal aunts and Alan's father had PhDs. Erik, Alan's older brother, was classically gifted. From a young age, anything Erik set out to do, he excelled at. Alan, indeed, seemed to have a rosy future in store for him. But Fate gave Alan both a trauma and a birth defect, each of which lay hidden for years.

The sun was shining brightly on a spring afternoon when the phone rang. I'd been required to have a physical exam before beginning a new job as a part-time ESL teacher - a job that, after several changes in career, I'd truly fallen in love with. When the voice on the phone told me I was pregnant, I was absolutely stunned. I'd had to take fertility pills to become pregnant with my first son, Erik. How was it possible for me to be pregnant again now without even trying? My thoughts swirled.

My first son, Erik, had cried nonstop for the first three months of his life and was now a very active and difficult five-year old. In addition to my new career as an ESL teacher, I'd accepted a summer job as a secretary in a day camp. I'd also applied for a master's degree program in teaching English as a second language.

Money was always tight. My husband at the time, a research scientist, was dependent on government grants and had previously been out of work for a full year. A new baby would definitely not make life any easier. Was it any wonder that the woman on the phone sensed my dismay and asked, *"Isn't that good news?"*

My immediate response was, "No."

The conversation ended with our scheduling an appointment with the OB/GYN.

Within just a few minutes, though, I began to feel the anticipation of having a new baby in our lives. Erik wouldn't grow up as an only child, and I'd always known how deeply my mother wished she'd had siblings. My husband, Roger, and I had always said that if we had a second child, it would be when our first child was in kindergarten, and Erik would be by the time the baby was born. By then, Erik would be independent enough not to feel pushed aside by a newborn sibling.

I called my supervisor at work the next day, and she readily agreed to grant me maternity leave. The job in the camp and the master's program were scrubbed with little regret; it would just be too hard to do it all. The next step was a visit to the OB/GYN covered by our health insurance.

When I arrived at the OB/GYN's office, I was astounded to find that a "termination" had been scheduled. While I had been less than excited on the phone, I had definitely not asked for an abortion. I had really only needed a few moments to get my bearings after receiving the news, but the cracks in the healthcare system were becoming visible. How could such a major decision about care, and about a life, be made without the patient's expressed consent or even consultation?

I informed the receptionist that I had every intention of keeping my baby, and we agreed that my appointment that day would be for a regular prenatal exam instead. At the beginning of that prenatal exam, the doctor asked me when I had last menstruated.

"You can't go by my menstrual cycle," I explained, *"I can go months without having my period."*

But the doctor insisted, and I told her when I'd last had my period. At that point, the doctor informed me that the fetus was close to three months. Because of my age (37), she advised scheduling an amniocentesis (amnio). Roger and I drove into Manhattan to Beth Israel Hospital where a sonogram of the fetus was taken before the amnio procedure. Viewing the image on the screen, the technician informed us that the fetus was not yet three months, and we'd have to come back.

When I returned to the OB/GYN for a follow-up visit and told her about the sonogram, she said, *"Oh, I must have mistaken your fibroid for the fetus."* Apparently, she'd discovered a fibroid (a benign tumor of muscular and fibrous tissues) during the original internal exam, a fibroid that neither she nor my previous gynecologist had ever mentioned.

"Could that affect the pregnancy?" I asked.

"Well," she said, *"it could cause a miscarriage."*

First, medical professionals had decided on a course of action (an abortion) that the patient (me) neither wanted nor asked for. As I'd soundly rejected the notion of an abortion, it should have been clear that I wanted to keep my baby. What effect could mentioning the possibility of a miscarriage have other than to terrify me? Was there something she could have told me about preventing or minimizing the risk of miscarriage? My experiences with this medical office were casting a terrible pall over my pregnancy. I put on my clothes and left, determined to find another OB/GYN.

The attitude of the new OB/GYN seemed better, and I soon had an amnio that revealed no problems. We learned I was having another boy. This, too, was a surprise. My mother-in-law already had four grandsons. Based on the law of averages, I was fully expecting my second child to be a girl and was momentarily disappointed. Upon deliberation, however, I thought having a second son was good news. Having a boy meant I wouldn't have to deal with the mood swings of teen girls—or so I thought.

Despite the rocky start, the pregnancy was otherwise uneventful. On some occasions, breathing became difficult because my uterus was tipped and pressing on my lungs. No big deal. Especially not in comparison to the joy I'd feel when lying on the couch, feeling the baby kick. This was a new experience for me because Erik had not been very active in my womb.

Several hours before dawn on January 30th 1986, I felt what seemed to be a particularly strong kick, and my water broke. This was also a new experience for me as my water had not broken during my first pregnancy. I couldn't believe how much water there was, and the drop of blood I spied was particularly frightening. Roger called his sister to come stay with Erik, and I went up to Erik's room to tell him I'd be back soon with his baby brother. With things at home well in hand, Roger pulled our Chevy Vega out of the garage and we were off to Syosset Hospital on Long Island.

At one point during labor, I was given oxygen because of "fetal distress." In later years, that fetal distress and the constant heartburn I experienced during my pregnancy would seem to have been harbingers of the "distress" that would eventually be the dominant theme in Alan's life, while heartache would be my life's theme. But at first, there were no signs that a troubled future lay ahead.

We came home from the hospital to big brother Erik and a house filled with love. For some reason, we started to call Alan "A.J.," his initials. He was such a good baby! He slept in a bassinet beside the living room couch so that we wouldn't have to move Erik out of his room. To my utter amazement, Alan slept through the night! As the weeks passed, he actually cooed. If he made sounds of discomfort when lying in his crib, we'd "shookle" him, putting a hand on his back and gently shaking him. He'd also be soothed if someone made the sound of an owl – hoo hoo.

When I was home, I would put Alan in one of those inclined baby seats in the bassinet and wheel him into whichever room I was in. He would grasp a stuffed animal, wave it around or suck on it, and be content so long as he could watch me. He did have one cranky period every day. He'd have a bottle around 10 P.M. and, an hour later, he'd be fussing and crying. If he had a second bottle, he'd sleep until about 7 A.M. Pure Heaven! But maybe he'd get too fat? The pediatrician laughed when I told her the situation.

"He's a tanker," she said. "He tanks up for the night and sleeps until morning."

I returned to work when Alan was only three weeks old. Our financial situation demanded that I work, and I was fortunate enough to have a part-time teaching job at the local high school. We were also very fortunate to find a loving and dependable woman who came to the house to take care of Alan every day. I was only gone from 10 A.M. to 3 P.M, but it hurt to be away from my baby and I now wonder if my absence affected Alan.

Did my return to work limit the all-important bonding between mother and child thereby affecting Alan's ability to feel secure? Psychologists tell us that early bonding plays a critical role in the "long-term mental health and resilience of children."[16] At that time, there was no reason to wonder about it.

Alan was an active child who could only be deemed "normal." He did the things little boys do at the appropriate age. In "psycho-speak," he reached "developmental milestones" right on target.

Before he was a year old, Alan started to walk and, just days later, he said his first word. He was looking out of the living room window while his dad was holding him, and he uttered "gark," which was the way he said "dark." This first word was followed quickly by "shoe," a strange choice of a second word. By the time Alan was 18 months old, he was speaking in complete sentences. Before he started school, he had learned to swim. He had also mastered both the bicycle and the scooter. The only developmental milestone that was not on target was tying his shoelaces, which he didn't accomplish until he was seven.

One of Alan's great childhood loves was a little pillow with a blue and white ruffled border. Every night, Alan lay his head upon it and touchthe ruffle around the edge. When the pillow became worn, my mother – Gram'Bea (short for Grandma Beatrice) – made a yellow and white checked pillow case for it. Alan was very unhappy with the new pillowcase, and I cut the two ends open so that he could continue to feel the ruffle while I read bedtime stories to him.

Although he very much liked the story *Jack and the Beanstalk*, Alan hated when I intoned *"Fe fi fo fum, I smell the blood of an Englishman"* in a scary voice. Looking back, it seems fitting that Alan enjoyed the story of a boy whose life was bettered by a climb up into the sky above. He also loved *The Pussycat Tiger*, a Golden Book about a tiger cub who worries that he will never be as big and strong as his father. Of course, the cub does grow up to be just like his dad. I think Alan identified with the cub. He, too, yearned to occupy the world of his father and brother as an equal. And perhaps the book helped spur Alan's lifelong love of animals.

Eventually, the woman who had cared for Alan from the time he was three weeks old found a different job. Another wonderful lady who lived just blocks away agreed to come in every morning to get Erik ready for school and take A.J. back to her house. She'd then pick Erik up after school, along with her own children. In her lovely musical Irish brogue, Mrs. Kelly frequently called A.J. "the best boy," and she'd go on to say, *"You could take him to the White House, he's so good."*

Basically, *life* was good. The boys and I would often sing, *"With two kids in the yard, life used to be so hard."* Alan loved singing. He'd sing while riding in the shopping cart at the market. Once, his rendition of *Frosty the Snowman* elicited the comment, *"At least someone has the holiday spirit."* At the playground, he'd sit on a swing that looked like a horse, swinging so high my heart would be in my mouth, all the while singing *"Jeremiah was a bullfrog, was a good friend of mine. I never understood a single word he said, but he helped me drink my wine."* His love of music and singing continued throughout his life as did the twinkle in his eyes and his impish smile. Behind that smile, however, was a little boy beginning to lose his way.

Alan was the most mellow of children during these preschool years. At the same time, Erik was the "squeaking wheel that got the oil." Alan could entertain himself for hours with his G.I. Joe toys or with video games.

Erik, on the other hand, constantly needed help with homework or needed to be chauffeured to an activity, or simply wanted attention. The best place for Erik to get the attention he craved was at the dinner table.

At dinner, the boys' father would always discuss science and technology with Erik. Discussions about physics and computers were common, which left Alan and me totally out of the conversation. Neither Alan's father nor his brother ever really gave Alan the floor, and, if they did let him speak, they were often dismissive of his contribution. Perhaps this explains Alan's reluctance to join the dinner group, and his preference for playing solitary video games.

When Alan graduated preschool, he decided he wanted a parakeet as a graduation gift, and he chose a vivid green one. He named the parakeet "Limey, the Green Rocketeer," after the hero of the 1991 Walt Disney movie *The Rocketeer*.

Poor little Limey was with us just one day. Perhaps this was the first of the traumas that would mark Alan's early years. We brought Limey's body back to the pet shop, where Alan chose a blue parakeet. He named this one Rama Lama Ding Dong from an old rock song that he loved to sing, and we called the bird Rama, for short. Rama lived with us for about eight years and actually learned to talk. Believe it or not, he could say *"I need a vacation, let me out."*

When Rama started to appear sick one day, Alan wanted me to take him to a doctor. Knowing that parakeets don't usually live long and doubting a vet could treat him, I got some medicine at the pet store. Rama refused to take it even when I tried to sneak it to him on a piece of lettuce, his favorite treat. He held the lettuce in his beak and shook it till the medicine came off. We were all devastated when we found Rama lying on the floor of his cage one morning. Rama was buried in the backyard in a very formal funeral ceremony, which included Erik's playing taps on his trumpet. Alan would love animals throughout his life.

During the summer after preschool, Erik and Alan went to the school district's Summer Recreation Program. It was there at the age of four that Alan made his stage debut. In the talent show, he did a comedy routine starting off with, "You can call me A.J., or you can call me Alan, but don't call me late for dinner." He ended with a famous line from the *Terminator* movie he so loved. Walking off the stage he turned back briefly, intoning "I'll be baahk" in a near perfect imitation of Arnold Schwarzenegger.

Ever so quickly, it was time for Alan to start kindergarten. I'd like to say "he became a student," but that term would never quite fit him. In kindergarten, he chose to be called Alan instead of A.J. On the first day, he happily ran into the room to be with the other children. He already knew some of them from the park and would soon be a participant in the ritual of playdates. But kindergarten days were not halcyon days.

In October of that school year, school officials informed me that the school's pre-admission testing conducted in April had revealed that Alan had a small motor skill deficit. Small or fine motor skills refer to the movements made using the small muscles in hands, wrists and fingers. Because these skills are used for just about every school task , from holding a pencil and writing neatly to using scissors or other tools for arts and crafts, they are critical to a student's early success and development.

Alan's motor skill deficit explained why he'd had so much trouble learning to tie his shoelaces and presaged some of the academic difficulties that were to come.

If school officials had let us know the results of the pre-admission testing earlier, we could have worked on helping Alan overcome the deficit months before school started. Instead, his school career began with frustration caused by his difficulties holding a crayon, cutting paper, and learning to write letters.

These difficulties didn't stop Alan from being creative, though. One of his kindergarten drawings is his interpretation of our morning ritual in which I'd wake him with a kiss and a hearty, "Up and at 'em." The drawing shows him sitting up in bed with the words, "Up and Adam" written in a bubble above his head.

When Alan was in kindergarten, his father became very ill. A biliary obstruction caused Roger, my husband and Alan's father, to turn yellow, truly yellow. I wouldn't have believed it if I hadn't seen it. Roger had an endoscopy, and the doctor who gave me the initial diagnosis said, "He either has scar tissue from his gallbladder surgery or it's cancer." No softening the blow by saying it might be a tumor.

"Cancer," he said, the disease that so terrified my parents that they couldn't even say the word. They had always referred to as "the big C." Once again, a doctor's way with words was caused distress, this time, for all of us. When Roger was scheduled for surgery, Erik wrote in school of his fear for his dad, choosing to express rather than repress his emotions, but Alan began his lifelong habit of keeping his darkest fears within him.

Each day, I visited Roger in Doctor's Hospital in New York City, traveling about 45 minutes each way to and from our house in Nassau County on Long Island. At this time, Alan was becoming increasingly difficult at home. Ms. Kelley's "best boy" began giving his Gram'Bea a hard time about everything.

Soon, Roger returned home following a successful biliary surgery, but, by then Alan had adopted the line, "Why should I?" in response to every request, a line that remained with him for several years.

I felt that Alan's difficult attitude was a reaction to his father's seeming disappearance and the concurrent prolonged absences of his mother. Perhaps this is also when his lifelong fear of abandonment began. Dark brushstrokes would increasingly appear on the canvas of Alan's life. The best boy was disappearing into the darkness, and a troubled youth was emerging.

Several months later, Roger's mother, Alan's paternal grandmother, passed away. Alan took her death very hard, crying himself to sleep on several nights. Somewhere around this time, he also started wetting the bed despite having been toilet trained for quite some time.

We would put two sets of sheets on the bed, complete with a second mattress cover and a plastic tablecloth in between the sheets. In the middle of the night, I'd hear him call for me on the intercom, go upstairs to his room, change his pajamas and pull off the top set of sheets. Did I reproach him or yell at him for bed-wetting? I have no recollection; I was practically sleepwalking. How I yearn to know that I was compassionate or at least tolerant…

About a year after Alan's paternal grandmother passed, his maternal grandmother – Gram'Bea – began to lose her sight. When she died almost ten years later at the age of 86, she was legally blind from a combination of acute closed angle glaucoma, retinal hemorrhage, and dry macular degeneration. Alan and his Gram'Bea were very close, and I am sure he was deeply affected by her loss of vision. So many unsettling events in the life of one small boy! Were illness, death, and blindness traumatic experiences for a five-year old? If so, did the traumas contribute to his acting out?

When Alan was in first grade, his teacher had him assigned to a special reading class because he couldn't read. When the reading teacher met with him, she was surprised: he could read – and quite well. He simply refused to do so until *he* wanted to. He was also constantly being criticized for his illegible handwriting, and he hated doing homework, which took time away from his playing video games.

First grade is a child's first real school experience, including a full day of learning and the homework that follows. At this time, lifelong patterns are established. For Alan, this meant a lifetime of hatred of school. Toward the end of first grade, I had to carry him down the stairs from his bedroom and fight to get him dressed and into the car. That continued until he got too big to carry. Instead, screaming and threats started our days.

By the end of first grade, Alan's handwriting was so bad that we were advised to get an occupational therapist to work with him. This was not a recommendation that I leaped to fulfill as my older son's experiences led me to be distrustful of the "professionals" in our school district.

When Erik was in elementary school, teachers frequently complained about his speaking out of turn — loudly. The principal even suggested we see a child psychologist. When Erik was in middle school and Alan was in first grade, Erik was placed in honors classes. Everything changed. Finally challenged and no longer needing to vent his boredom, Erik became a model student. Considering these circumstances, it shouldn't be surprising that I distrusted the judgment of school personnel. Little did I know how their poor judgment would color our lives in years to come.

My distrust led me to find a private occupational therapist to independently evaluate Alan. She concurred that he had some deficits. Since hiring a therapist ourselves would have been prohibitively expensive, we decided to have Alan classified as a special education student so that he could receive occupational therapy services in school and at no cost to us.

The occupational therapist that the school hired to provide the in-school services asked that a slant board be purchased for Alan to use in class. The tilted board provides support for the wrist and arm so that a person can write more legibly. The occupational therapist expected Alan to use this board whenever he had to write or draw.

The school district had used taxpayer dollars to hire a specialist to make recommendations on Alan's behalf, but those around Alan were either unwilling or incapable of following them. For example, Alan's regular classroom teacher was clueless about the slant board's use. One day when I dropped Alan off at school, she actually asked *me* what she should do with it.

On top of that, having the slant board on his desk during his regular class time was akin to erecting a billboard proclaiming, "Alan is different. Alan can't do things other students can do," in huge letters. Having the slant board made Alan feel especially different from other kids. If there's one thing children don't want, it's to feel different. Like pups in a litter, children need to feel that they are no different than any other child and that they belong to the group. If not, they feel insecure and anxious. Here was the first inkling that the system was likely to prescribe a treatment that was worse than the disease.

In addition to regular meetings with the occupational therapist, Alan was assigned to the special education resource room for part of each school day. Because a classroom teacher can't give individualized attention to each of 20 to 30 students, schools label the most problematic students as "special" so that they can get more personalized help in smaller class settings and resource rooms.

People were always absolutely stunned to hear that Alan was a "special ed" student. His verbal skills were extraordinary, and he was clearly a smart boy. I had to constantly explain that Alan was a special ed student because of a physical rather than a cognitive handicap.

Once again, Alan was being made to feel different from his peers. As one psychologist put it, "When we find ourselves in situations where we are the "out- group" or in an environment in which we feel like an outsider, we use our mental energy to monitor for threats, leaving fewer resources for higher cognitive processes."[17]

Throughout his school years, Alan's academic progress would continually be was hampered by "solutions" that increased his insecurities. Although the reports from pre-school had always said Alan "worked and played well with others," he began to have angry outbursts that continued as he got older.

He once kicked a locker in the hallway of his elementary school. On another occasion, when Alan's two best friends told him they wouldn't come to his Halloween party, he kicked the door at one of their houses. When he went to a summer recreation program, he got into physical altercations with one particular boy every year and would end up being suspended for two days each time. At home, he'd slam or throw toys that didn't operate as he wanted them to.

I did everything I could think of to get him to control his temper. Time-outs never worked. I'd put him in his little chair facing the door and he'd get up over and over again. I started trying to convince him that angry outbursts wouldn't accomplish anything.

I'd coach him to *"walk softly and carry a big stick,"* trying to make him be like the actor Gary Cooper — the strong silent type. *"Stand up as tall and straight as you can; take a step in, look down your nose, and talk tough. Let people know you aren't afraid, and you won't take anything from them."* Little did I know how well Alan would learn this lesson. Several times in later years, I'd see him take that stance in confrontations, even with me.

In resource room, Alan was angry because someone was always looking over his shoulder, checking his work, and making comments on his abilities (or lack thereof). He also experienced frustration because the resource room teachers did not always help him achieve his goals.

In one meeting, I was told that Alan couldn't use scissors. I pointed out that he was left-handed and asked if he was using a left-handed scissors. "When he asks for it," was the answer. Expecting a student who exhibits issues with authority and a lack of self confidence to reach out for help, especially in relation to the physical "disability" that placed him in the special needs situation in the first place, seems ludicrous. These are supposed to be special needs education professionals?

In second grade, students started learning to write essays, but Alan couldn't produce one that met the teacher's requirements. When I was told that Alan "couldn't write an essay," my sense that the "professionals" were less than sterling only increased. Weren't the educators in the resource room aware that Alan had small motor skill difficulty, including a mild tremor that the occupational therapist called a "concentration tremor"? Wasn't it obvious that writing was physically difficult for him?

This physical problem certainly made it difficult for him to create essays – it made it difficult for him to write anything at all, as evidenced by his poor penmanship. I had to remind both the classroom teacher and the resource room teacher about the physical difficulties and suggested that he use a computer for writing essays.

While on the surface my idea seemed to have merit, I was informed by the teachers that the idea had failed. We all should have realized that he wouldn't be able to write an essay on a computer: he didn't know how to type! It was laborious to type sentences or paragraphs, let alone essays, when each key had to be hunted for and pecked at. Desperately searching for a solution, I then suggested that he be permitted to tape record his "writings." That didn't work either. I was told he "played with the tape recorder buttons."

Why did the professionals tend to throw their hands up in defeat and simply dismiss the student? Why was it that the only one looking for alternatives was the concerned parent? Shouldn't the educators who were trained to work with "special" students have been able to recognize and deal with these problems? Couldn't they figure out a solution for what was a relatively common problem – a child with motor skill deficits that couldn't correctly use a writing implement? You would have thought it was 1930, not 1990.

Despite all of Alan's problems in school, he continued to make friends with other boys in the neighborhood and was an active participant in the local scouting troop. In all the things Alan did, it was obvious that he yearned for recognition, and when he received it, his joy was palpable.

One incident occurred when he was only about eight years old. Alan and a friend were walking near our local park, and they saw an elderly woman on the ground by her house. Alan ran to her and discovered that she could not get up, so he quickly found an adult in the park who called for an ambulance.

Alan stayed with the woman until the ambulance came and later learned that she had broken her hip. When several people, including the firefighters who arrived on the scene, praised him for his concern and quick-thinking, Alan glowed. He couldn't wait to tell Roger, Erik, and me the story. He also wrote about it in a writing exercise in school: *"I like to help seniors because when I help someone it feels good inside like when I helped an old lady when she fell and broke her hip."*

For once, Alan was receiving attention for having done something good instead of criticism for having not lived up to expectations. But at school, Alan's behaviors seemed to garner only negative comments and criticism.

Alan had trouble completing tasks and frequently misplaced materials. Don't ask how many wrist bracelets we bought to hold his lunch money and how many of those bracelets simply disappeared. His classroom teacher was absolutely convinced that he had attention deficit hyperactivity disorder (ADHD). Years of psychological and psychiatric evaluations and scores of drug trials were about to begin.

School district officials made an appointment for Alan to be evaluated by a psychiatrist. Alan's father and I went with Alan to the consult. When we arrived, we learned that the school had reported to the psychiatrist that Alan *"is learning disabled."* It's interesting that the school reported that *prior* to the evaluation, perhaps setting Alan up for what is termed "confirmation bias." One psychologist explains this bias as "People are prone to believe what they want to believe."[18] Would this prejudice end up coloring the results of the evaluation?

The school's "diagnosis" was apparently based on his *"fine motor skill problems, particularly in handwriting as well as opening his string cheese."* It sounds almost comical that "string cheese" was singled out to produce a label of "learning disabled," as if difficulties opening packaging were emblematic of a serious mental handicap. In any event, small motor skill deficits and learning disabled are not synonymous.

The elementary school also reported that *"Alan is inattentive and lacks motivation. These complaints have been present for the last 3 years."* In addition, it was pointed out that Alan's *"attention is variable. He has a lack of self-control and talks out of turn."* This is not uncommon among little boys in school, but usually isn't a reason to send a child for psychological evaluation.

School personnel also saw that Alan "is easily frustrated. He becomes angry and aggressive [when he becomes frustrated]." Yes, Alan was often frustrated in life and expressed it with anger. Did anyone stop to question what was making such a young child so angry?

Looking back with the knowledge I've gained doing research for this book, it's clear to me that Alan was displaying the hyperarousal symptoms associated with PTSD, which include feeling irritable, being impulsive, having nightmares, and angry outbursts. "This can lead to severe bouts of depression and may manifest with self-destructive behaviors…"[19]

Shouldn't a mental health professional have considered that Alan was evidencing the "disruptive, disrespectful, or destructive" symptoms of children with PTSD and looked into that possibility?

Following the consultation, we received a copy of the psychiatrist's report. It was surprising to see the comment that there are "no sleep problems," a point supposedly gleaned from his conversations with Alan's father and me.

Actually, Alan had long been having problems with insomnia, and it's impossible to believe that neither of us mentioned it. I distinctly remember telling several teachers that I felt Alan's insomnia was his biggest problem: lack of sleep always interferes with concentration and usually makes people very cranky.

About a year after this consultation, Alan underwent an intensive day of evaluation at North Shore University Hospital's Neurobehavioral Clinic. Alan received a diagnosis of attention-deficit disorder, predominantly inattentive rather than hyperactive type. This label is based on an individual's chronic inability to pay attention but is not characterized by extreme activity or impulsivity.

It was also determined that Alan had oppositional defiant disorder. This behavior disorder is marked by uncooperative, negative, and irritable behavior.

It was also noted that Alan had *"some excellent skills notably in word knowledge, information, and reading."* One suggestion was that Alan be allowed *"extended testing time to allow [him] to fully express his vast knowledge."* This option was available throughout Alan's education, but he constantly refused to avail himself of it. In Alan's mind, extended testing time was another sign of his "stupidity," inferiority, or just plain difference from others.

The report from that day also reads:

This was an alert, pleasant boy whose fund of knowledge seemed to be appropriate for his age. He was able to remain seated in one place and was not fidgety. His attention span was adequate but his organization skills were poor. His mathematical and reading skills seem to be adequate… performance IQ was 17 points lower than his verbal IQ… This is an 8-year-old with predominant difficulty in his visual motor, fine motor tasks and attention span as well as some frustration which may have been related to the above. He does meet all the classical criteria for attention deficit, hyperactivity disorder which would warrant use of a psychostimulant medication.

In schools, a ten-point disparity between performance and verbal IQ is usually regarded as evidence of a learning disability. Given this evidence and the other evaluation results, Ritalin was prescribed.

Recent statistics reveal that "males are almost three times more likely to be diagnosed with ADHD than females"[20] and more than 60 percent of children being treated for ADHD are prescribed stimulants such as Ritalin.[21] Use of the drug is so widespread that I remember reading a *New York Times* article that suggested Tom Sawyer and Huckleberry Finn would be prescribed Ritalin if they were in school today.

Alan's father and I were against using medication. We didn't even let our boys eat or drink anything with artificial sweeteners for fear of long-term effects, and we were now supposed to start pumping our son full of pills?

Eventually, we relented due to our frustration and fatigue, and because we were assured that the pills would work as a diagnostic tool: if Alan's ability to concentrate and perform in school improved, it would be clear that he really did have ADHD. If the medicine didn't work, alternative diagnoses would be explored.

The drug didn't seem to affect Alan's ability to concentrate. Even if it had, it wasn't worth the side effects: Ritalin caused Alan to become withdrawn, and he started exhibiting signs of depression. The drug trial was stopped.

Around this time, Alan started to go to group therapy sessions for social skills and anger management. The program did help him with anger and impulse control. He learned not to voice his resistance at the "wrong times," but would return from school and, in later years, from work and complain bitterly about teachers and supervisors who picked on him or about their "stupidity."

In spite of Alan's improved ability to deal with frustration and anger, school continued to be a struggle. His dislike of school was fully ingrained.

Every day was a battle to get Alan just to go to school. Every morning he would stay in the shower way too long and be late to school. When he came home, the battle shifted to trying to get him to do his homework. Often, he'd forget to take any homework he had managed to do. He had now begun to write essays with great imagination and creativity. Still, there were teachers who chose to harp on his terrible handwriting and spelling and failed to applaud his creativity. This lack of recognition from teachers hurt Alan deeply, so he pulled his head deeper into his hooded sweatshirts, tuned out, and shut down.

Were teachers focusing on Alan's weaknesses in response to the labels he'd been given? Why were they failing to applaud his strengths? His verbal IQ, which measures cognitive ability, was 118, which was in the 88th percentile, meaning only 22 percent of his peers had higher IQs.

The school seemed to focus on his performance IQ, which measures ability to physically manipulate objects by assembling or arranging them. Alan's performance IQ was 17 points lower than his verbal IQ.

On achievement tests in reading, he scored in the 98th percentile. His cognitive ability was in the 82nd percentile. His math skills were in the 74th percentile. Yet Alan constantly brought home report cards with failing grades — so much potential, so little actualization. Alan reminded me of a Peanuts cartoon in which a character says, "potential is a terrible burden."

While Alan's verbal skills, creativity and potential motivated some teachers and the special education staff at school to work to get him on track, to Alan, these people were just "in his face."

Eventually a trial of Dexedrine was started. Like Ritalin, Dexedrine is a stimulant that sometimes can help increase attention span, control impulsive behavior, and reduce hyperactivity in children. Again, the side effects made it impractical to continue the medication.

My recollection of Alan chattering away in the back seat of the car as his dad and I looked at each other in amazement is vivid to this day. The Dexedrine had turned Alan into a non-stop motor mouth. How was that going to help him function in school? Furthermore, it worsened his insomnia, which made him more belligerent and cranky. His teacher said she would rather he be fidgety. When I asked her, "What am I going to do with him?" she replied, "Just love him." I did, but it simply was never enough.

Love, pills, labels — nothing was helping Alan realize his potential or be happy.

My frustration wasn't helped when one of the psychiatrists explained that the diagnoses of various mental illnesses were basically made by checking off a laundry list of symptoms. If a patient checks a majority of the systems on any list, the diagnosis is made, or at least the label is applied. A system like this doesn't seem either scientific or objective.

Symptoms that one practitioner checks off may not be seen by another and may not be seen in all situations. People are the sum total of many parts—cognition, emotion, physiology—and the relationship of these parts is constantly in flux, responding differently to different people, situations, and environments. Can any label or even combination of labels possibly contain all of that?

Under the circumstances, it's not surprising that Alan suffered from low self-esteem. Continuously shuttled from resource room to school counselor to therapist to group therapy, Alan was constantly being reminded that something was not as it should be; that he was somehow different.

It didn't help that his brother was gifted. One school counselor commented that Alan had said, "I wish I had my brother's brain" and acknowledged being jealous of his brother. All through the years to come, Alan would adore his big brother and yearn for Erik's respect. I'd watch the two of them at holiday dinners, noticing that whenever Alan said something, he'd glance at Erik out of the corner of his eye to gauge Erik's reaction.

I may have added to Alan's emotional problems when he was 12, as I decided to leave his father. At that time, my mother was legally blind, frail, and forgetful. Fortunately, she had moved into an apartment very close to our house, and I was able to help her in many ways. Unfortunately, taking care of a mother, two sons, and a demanding husband was more than I could deal with.

As I neared 50, it became clear that if my life was ever going to change, I had to change it.

Erik had left home to attend college, and Alan and I moved into a one-bedroom apartment in the same building that my mother lived in. It was walking distance from Alan's dad's house, which was ideal since we had joint custody. It also meant that we'd be living right across the street from Alan's best friend, which I'm sure was his primary motivation in asking to live in "Gram'Bea's building."

By this time, Alan's small motor deficit and even ADHD were the least of his problems. Psychological issues were now at the crux of the IEP—individualized educational plan — that school personnel drafted and kept revising.

As time passed, Alan's classification as a special education student would run the gamut from learning disabled to "multiply handicapped." At one point, we'd been asked to approve the classification of "emotionally disturbed" but refused.

Any label we give a child is harmful to the child's sense of self, but "emotionally disturbed" was a label with a truly devastating sound. Once a person is labeled, he believes himself to *be* what the label says he is. This is obviously detrimental to self-esteem. Moreover, people treat others according to their perceived notions and prejudices surrounding the labels. This is not what I wanted for my baby.

At the end of 7th grade, a private psychiatrist we were seeing diagnosed Alan with Dysthymia, sometimes referred to as mild, chronic depression. "Childhood depression," he pointed out, "is often misdiagnosed as ADHD."

This psychiatrist saw what others had missed, perhaps prodded by the information that Alan's maternal tree had a history of depression, and that his maternal grandfather (my father) had been hospitalized for the condition. The doctor prescribed Zoloft, which Alan took for a short period of time. More labels. More pills. Still no real answers.

Why was an intelligent, creative, loving child not functioning in school? Why was anger frequently his way of dealing with difficulties? And on those occasions when things were going well, why did Alan find a reason to walk away? Over and over, counselors and teachers kept asking why he "sabotaged" himself.

Without any real answers, the school district repeatedly turned to more testing. In 1999, when Alan was 13, he underwent an extensive battery of tests as part of the New York State mandate that special education students be re-evaluated every three years.

The testing occurred about a year after I had separated from Alan's father and a little more than a year after Erik had started college and moved out. For any child, these events would constitute an upheaval with emotional consequences, which Alan was clearly experiencing. He told the tester, "I didn't leave my father, my mother left him."

It had never been my intention for Alan to "leave his father." We lived within walking distance from Alan's dad precisely so that Alan could go there whenever he wanted. His dad and I had agreed that Alan would spend weekends with his father in his childhood home.

If I had visions of father and son making up for lost time and enjoying each other's company on those weekends, those visions disappeared quickly. Alan become more and more reluctant to go to his dad's. It would take five more years for me to learn why he hated going to that house.

At the same testing session in 1999, Alan was asked what he would want if he could have three wishes and he responded: "Make mom a little less oppositional. Have a perfect American family. Have a lot of money so I don't have to worry."

Obviously, my constant worry about money had been passed along to Alan. I received no child support from his father until our divorce was finalized about a year after I left, and I had been working several part-time jobs to provide us with food, clothing, and shelter. That wasn't a burden Alan should have shared.

As for my being "oppositional"—how telling that Alan was beginning to use psychological jargon at a young age. It demonstrated how inundated he was by mental health services and evaluations, and how the process of labeling him had led him to label others in the same manner.

In truth, it was hard to "be less oppositional" with Alan. He'd take a shower before school and not get out no matter how much I yelled. He was always late to school. He'd disappear when he had orthodontist appointments, and I'd yell at him for that. I'd fight with him to stop playing video games and go to bed, to do his homework, to pick his clothes up off the floor or to put his dishes in the sink. Obviously, my being oppositional accomplished nothing for either of us.

By the end of middle school, the school psychologist reported that "Alan presented as more and more depressed as the year progressed and admitted to having suicidal ideations." These were terrifying words for a parent to hear!

Alan was in and out of private counseling, but he didn't seem to connect with the therapists and went inconsistently. He began antidepressant medication at the end of the school year but discontinued it after complaints to the psychiatrist about side effects. One of which was a diminished ability to feel much of anything, which may have led to at least one incident of Alan cutting himself. Although most teens who self-mutilate do so in an attempt to release emotional pain, others harm themselves because it allows them to feel something other than numbness.

A retest of Alan's IQ around this time revealed that his verbal IQ had grown to a "Very Superior" rating of 132. His performance IQ was 100, "Average," and he scored consistently above the 12th grade level across all subject areas even though he was only in eighth grade. Sadly, social/emotional testing indicated:

"[Alan] is a depressed youngster who appears to be overwhelmed by his own emotions. He has completely shut down academically and emotionally in school... Although Alan participates on team sports, he doesn't have the commitment needed to follow through for an entire season... Alan has been known to become easily distracted and displays inattentive behavior. His emotional needs seem to exacerbate these behaviors."

As Alan's emotional problems increasingly interfered with his ability to function in school, concern for him increased and that called for yet another medication. This time, it was the antidepressant Wellbutrin.

I wasn't surprised that Alan was being treated for depression. Both my father and my paternal aunt had been treated for it, so a genetic component was likely. Environment played a role, too. Alan was surrounded by overachieving family members: his father and a paternal aunt had PhDs, another paternal aunt was a best-selling author, his older brother was intellectually gifted, a talented trumpet player, and an exceedingly good-looking young man.

Alan never felt he could compete with these people, so he reverted to his old refrain of "Why should I?" whenever he was asked to do anything. If he didn't make an effort to do well, his failures could always be attributed to that lack of effort rather than to deficits within himself. His years as a special education student only furthered his lack of self-esteem.

It seemed that we were on a road that was leading deeper and deeper into darkness. At one point in his mid-teens, Alan took to his bed for a full month. Nothing I did or said could get him to go to school, meet friends, or come to the table. He ate meals in bed and did little else but sleep.

Every morning on my way to work, I'd hide every sharp implement I could find in fear that he'd attempt to take his life or resort to self injury to relieve his psychological pain.

Eventually, Alan got out of bed. Was it just boredom that drove him back into the world? Was he able to summon inner resources? Or did he run out of drugs? He had been prescribed Klonopin for his anxiety. This medication can also cause drowsiness. I now suspect that Alan was taking more than the prescribed dose so that he could sleep pretty much all the time. If I had only considered the possibility that he had a drug problem, maybe I could have done something to stave off disaster.

When Alan finally returned to school after his month in bed, the school district decided that he needed to be outplaced in a school that served special needs students. The first of these was Education and Assistance

Corporation (EAC). Here, classes were very small, sometimes one-on-one, and the pace was individualized.

Alan had a successful year there, even receiving a good attendance commendation. The school district, however, would not permit him to stay, saying it could not be a permanent placement. How sad and ironic that the first "treatment" that was prescribed for Alan that provided extraordinarily promising results was so summarily dismissed.

Subsequently, Alan was sent to a Board of Cooperative Educational Services (BOCES) school, which offers students a large variety of programs and services that would be prohibitively expensive for individual school districts to provide. Alan was assigned to BOCES' Center for Community Adjustment, which is always referred to as CCA probably because the full name has such an onerous ring to it.

In addition to small classes and teachers trained to work with emotionally, behaviorally, or developmentally disabled students, CCA provided group and one-on-one psychological therapy. Alan didn't love it—he still wore hoodies that obscured his face and his view of the world—but here he met friends who would be by his side forever.

Because our apartment was not in the school district Alan had been attending, I had to take Alan to his dad's house every morning to get the bus to CCA. Two other students from Alan's high school also took that bus to CCA—Christine and Daniel. Alan had known and been friends with Daniel since elementary school, but hadn't known Christine before. At this time, Alan also met Adrianna, a good friend of Christine's but not a student at CCA.

Christine was a pretty and outspoken girl who soon captured Alan's interest. But she also captured the interest of another classmate — Marquand. For some young men, this situation could have led to fisticuffs, but Marquand is a truly gentle man who told Alan, *"Hey, man, Christina obviously likes you, and you guys will probably be happy together."* From that moment on, Marquand and Alan were best friends, and Christine became the first of Alan's "long-term" romantic relationships.

Alan was a "serial monogamist." Each of his relationships lasted at least a year, and he didn't date at all in between those relationships. When he didn't have a girlfriend, he was miserable. His journal entry from the time he broke up with one of his girlfriends best reveals that misery:

"Everything I say to you has become a kind of pathetic, futile supplication. A broken man begging an absent god to spare him his trials. Your vacant silence rings in my ears like some long forgotten record, the hiss and pop of pitted vinyl a syncopation of breath and heartbeat."

The prospect of being alone terrified him. He desperately needed to feel loved; he was often clingy and asked if I loved him. Having a girlfriend was one of the ways he kept his fears of abandonment at bay and allowed him to express both his romantic and protective sides.

At CCA, Alan also met his forever friends Pete and Gary. Gary recalls:

"I remember in high school when I first met Pete and Alan, sitting at their lunch table for the first time, so terrified I would be judged by them, I hardly said a word. But then Alan came over to me and whispered 'Swamp-Ass' in my ear and had me laughing so hard. He was the kind of person who would say the most random things just to get a smile or a laugh out of people. Peter and Alan welcomed me like one of their own and from then on, our friendship began."

During Alan's teen years, I realized how well he had been listening to my talk about walking tall. Marquand tells the story of a girl he and Alan knew who was being harassed by the boy she was dating. Alan stepped into the scene with, "You got about two seconds to back up. Don't make me repeat myself." Alan was always quick to offer support to troubled friends. How often I'd hear him on the phone, helping friends through various crises, sometimes even repeating things *I'd* told him. His friend Gary says:

"With the three of us together, there was no obstacle we could not conquer, there was no problem that was left unsolved... When I was having a rough time in a relationship, Alan was always there, making a joke about it to make me smile and laugh. Peter and Alan would kidnap me from my house when I was depressed and didn't want to leave my room or my house.

They'd physically drag me out, and we would just go find an adventure. I'll never forget all the times I felt helpless and there were Peter and Alan to pick me back up."

Alan could certainly empathize with depression, but as the years passed, his anxiety seemed to become even more of a burden than his depression.

When I first left his father, I slept on a pull-out in the living room and Alan had the bedroom. Many nights, he would crawl into bed with me, nestle against my back, hug me, and hold my hand. I still feel Alan's hand holding mine when I lie on my side in bed. His actions and words constantly showed me how much he feared being left alone. On the day my cousin Steve told us he was moving to California to be with the man he loved, I found Alan crying at his computer.

"What's the matter? I know we were close with Steve, but not that close," I asked.

"If Steve can leave his son, you can leave me," Alan replied.

"There is no way I would ever leave you," I answered hugging him tightly.

Several years later, Andy, my boyfriend at the time, said I would pick Alan over him any day. Did Alan fear being abandoned because he felt unlovable? He never wanted anything more—or less—than to be loved and respected. Did he ever recognize that mostly he needed to love himself?

Love was the hallmark of Alan's life. That love extended to all people, especially to children, the elderly, and animals. Having been so very close to his two aging and infirm grandmothers, Alan had a special place in his heart for elderly women. In our apartment building, he was quick to open doors, help with packages, or find lost keys for the older women. Any time I meet one of the women in the building who knew him, she tells me about Alan's sweet nature and helpfulness.

Helping others made Alan feel good about himself, something he felt far too rarely. He also loved animals all his life and never forgot the *Pussycat Tiger* book.

Did Alan's hunger for approval recognize the unconditional love that pets give us? For years, he begged to have a cat. We weren't allowed to have pets in the apartment building we had moved to when I left his father, but we did go to the shelter a couple of times to look at the cats.

For Alan's 16th birthday, we visited the shelter again with the understanding that we would not bring home a cat; we were just going to look. There, in a corner of a large room filled with cat cages, was a white tabby with black and white on his head, back and tail. Not a kitten but not yet a full-grown cat, the tabby curiously sniffed at our fingers. We were able to take him to a closed-in area where he happily rubbed against us. His outgoing personality was readily apparent, and we both fell in love with him – so much for only looking.

Alan said if anyone objected to our having the cat, we'd say that Koshka was a "service cat." He'd read about Emotional Support Animals (ESA) whose presence helped people when they were emotionally distressed. The warm presence, cuddling, and unconditional love had been found helpful to those with emotional disorders including anxiety, depression, and post-traumatic stress disorder.

Over the years, Alan did find great comfort in lying with the cat on his belly. The cat's contented purring did soothe Alan at least temporarily. Alan's capacity for and desire to love and care for others didn't stop at people -- it extended to Koshka, too. At the slightest sign of distress, Alan would rush the cat to the vet. Perhaps Alan's desire to keep Koshka happy and contented was a compensation mechanism for his inability to control his own environment.

Sadly, Alan's intense capacity for love was frequently overshadowed by his depression and anger. Something had "turned" Mrs. Kelly's "best boy," and there was no pill on Earth that could change that. In spite of all the tests, all the psychologists, all the psychiatrists, and all the specialists, Alan's pain was too deep, too disguised, or too shameful to be revealed. And the professionals simply didn't recognize the signs.

Alan was 18 when he finally revealed the secret he had kept hidden from the time he was a small boy. I was sitting on the couch, watching TV, when Alan sat down and said, "I have something to tell you."

Alan revealed that he had been sexually abused by a young neighbor from the time he was about five until he was about 12 years old.

In spite of that revelation, the pieces of the puzzle that was Alan didn't come together in that instant. Over the coming years, I came to see and understand things that had been incomprehensible before I had that information. I eventually came to understand why Alan always voiced hatred for the town in which we lived, and why he hated to go back to his father's house: both of these locations were the scenes of his sexual abuse.

There is now absolutely no doubt in my mind that almost all of Alan's mental health problems could be attributed to PTSD. Alan had hidden his secret well, enduring shame and guilt, experiencing flashbacks and anger at circumstances that had robbed him of the sense of security that every child should have. So much damage had been done.

It would be wonderful to say that the revelation gave me and the mental health practitioners a new paint palette with which to change the canvas of Alan's life. Sadly, none of us were able to chip away the gloomy colors that had long ago hardened and dried, and we couldn't find a brush with which to cover that paint.

Alan continued to do poorly in school and continued to suffer from a lack of self esteem and a fear of abandonment. Often when sleep eluded him, he would call Adrianna who was always understanding and supportive. They'd talk until Alan began to feel drowsy.

When he did sleep, Alan suffered from terrifying nightmares. His insomnia made it very difficult for him to get up in the morning and go to work or school, and that difficulty often led to his quitting jobs or dropping out of school. In spite of everything — having not graduated high school with his peers, having had a rocky education, and rarely doing schoolwork — Alan managed to get his GED without even opening a review book.

I had been teaching English as a Second Language at the New York Institute of Technology (NYIT) for years. Now, with the GED, Alan could attend that college for free, which he did on and off for several semesters.

When he did attend, he did very well, even making the Dean's List one semester. Alan also had the third lead in the college's production of Shakespeare's *Love's Labour's Lost.* He was not only excellent in the part of Longaville, he even used the show as an opportunity to make an impression on his then-girlfriend Danielle. On opening night, she was sitting in the front row, and Alan approached her to deliver his lines about love directly to her. My boyfriend Andy was so impressed with Alan's performance that he tried to convince Alan to pursue acting as a career, saying that Alan reminded him of a young Marlon Brando. But this was not to be.

When Alan was about 25, a new love came into his life, and the shadows seemed to lift for a while. Christina (not the previously mentioned Christine) was a girl with whom he could have intellectual conversations and share his love of science, music, animals, and food.

Around the same time as this new-found romance, Alan was able to secure a job in information technology even though he had not yet earned his degree. He was employed by a man who had a small business fixing computers, and Alan was earning good money, which he very much enjoyed spending. He and Christina were starting to look for a place where they could live together. But Alan quit the job, saying that the owner kept delaying his pay. This was a significant problem since Alan had to lay out money to commute from Long Island to jobs in the city. Shortly after quitting the job, he and Christina broke up.

Alan sank into another very deep depression. He rarely went out of the house, spent almost all his time in bed, and started binge eating, a habit that continued until the time of his death. By the time he died, my little boy was so overweight that the autopsy report labeled him "obese." When we talked about this latest bout with depression, Alan said, *"If I can't ever be happy, why should I even try?"*

Did the damaged little boy believe that he didn't deserve happiness? Is that why he always sabotaged himself?

On top of it all, Alan told me that he was angry about his family's lack of respect for him. I tried to mollify him even though I was thinking, "You're in your late 20s and your mother is supporting you. Can it really be a surprise that your family doesn't respect you?"

I eventually realized that Alan's anger was directed at himself more than at his family. He vehemently hated not being independent and not being able to get past his anxiety and depression in order to become independent. It was always easier for him to complain about the way others—mostly me—treated him.

But Alan's world was not always black. When he was happy, he had the most wonderful smile—not broad or toothy but lit with a warmth that caused his eyes to twinkle. His laughter was often tinged with love and his love was just as often tinged with laughter. I see a perfect example of Alan's brand of humor in the note he wrote to me in a Mother's Day card when he was about 25:

"We've faced a lot together on this bumpy road of life. Despite the hardship and tears, the anxiety and fears, we have made it through. That's some cool shit!"

The child had an inimitable talent for making me laugh with tears in my eyes and making me cry with laughter on my lips.

Alan loved humor. Whether it was *Family Guy* or George Carlin, slapstick or political humor, Alan loved to laugh. For him, laughter was an antidote to pain.

"At the gym doing cardio. Trying to stave off the boredom by Facebooking. You late risers are ruining my workout. Make with the amusing idiocy already. You had ONE job. Smh."

His humor could be a bit macabre, even profane, at times:

"RIP Leslie Neilsen. I still think of you every time I get on a plane."

Or:

"Life getting tough just means the gods are afraid of your progress. ...You're on notice, gods."

Sometimes his humor was just plain silly. In a party invitation he wrote:

"Party night! Be there or be toroidal polyhedron."

Christina fondly remembers a Christmas they shared:

"Alan loved the Irish coffee my family made and [he] told my grandma he wanted to convert to Irishism."

He didn't just dish out the humor, he could poke fun at himself, too. He started to lose his hair in his 20s and put the following words in his father's mouth:

"Remember how you used to make fun of me for being bald? No, I'm not gonna make a joke. I'll let your mirror do that."

As important as laughter and love were to Alan, science may have meant even more to him. Totally convinced that the world needed to be a better place, he was equally sure that it could be achieved by following the precepts of science. He was passionate, for instance, on the issue of vaccinating children and appalled that any parent would consider avoiding the vaccines. To Alan, science was the cure for the ignorance and stupidity that he abhorred. One of his favorite quotes was by Bertrand Russell who said:

"One of the painful things about our time is that those who feel certainty are stupid, and those with any imagination and understanding are filled with doubt and indecision."

Despite Alan's understanding of the world picture—or perhaps because of it—he was plagued by doubts and fears.

One November night in 2011, Alan was in his room on his computer as usual. He'd recently started weight-lifting, which was to me a sign that he was in good spirits. I was watching TV and waiting for my boyfriend Andy to come home when the phone rang. Andy was downstairs, having trouble locking the car door, and he wanted Alan to come down to help. As soon as I told Alan what was up, he grabbed a screwdriver and headed out to assist. I returned to watching TV. Sometime later, the doorbell rang and I found myself facing three police officers with Andy in the background - but no Alan. I couldn't conceive of what was going on.

According to the officers, Alan had been online threatening to shoot himself, and one of his friends had called the police. When the police arrived on our street, Alan was curious about the ambulance and went over to see what was happening.

The police asked who he was and then told Alan to throw the screwdriver in the trash or they'd accuse him of coming at them with a weapon. They handcuffed him, put him in an ambulance, and took him to Nassau County Medical Center. The officers at my door wanted to search Alan's room for weapons.

Although I was beside myself with anxiety about my son, I asked if they needed a search warrant, but Andy told me to let them go ahead. I knew Alan had three rifles; he was very interested in target-shooting as his father had been. The police took the rifles, gave me a receipt and went on their way. I called Alan's dad and Andy and I rushed to the hospital.

The police had brought Alan in for mental observation; as it turned out, they may have saved his life. He was diagnosed with rhabdomyolysis. Known as RM and colloquially referred to as simply "rhabdo," this condition occurs when muscle tissue breaks down, leading to the release of toxic substances into the bloodstream. Severe RM can be fatal as it can lead to kidney failure, fatal heart rhythm and/or excess bleeding due to an inability to clot. In Alan's case, the condition might have been caused by extreme overexertion at the gym in combination with the various drugs he was taking. It is possible that he had been feeling lower than usual because of this physical condition.

Alan was on an IV for three days and had a "guard" for the first two days because of his suicide threat. He was also examined by a staff psychiatrist. Being kept "under guard" definitely didn't improve his mood, and when we checked out and his prescription medications weren't returned to him, I thought he would go ballistic.

One of the medications Alan was taking carried the risk of seizure if withdrawal was sudden; fortunately he was able to get more from his psychiatrist. Alan wondered what had become of the medications, which the police took when they searched his room. I wonder, too.

44

Why would they take and *not* return prescription drugs? Is it possible that the officers kept them for themselves? I'm sure I don't know, but the thought definitely entered both our minds.

Since this all happened around mid-term exam week, and Alan had missed several days of school, he decided to drop out that semester. It was becoming a pattern—he'd go to school for a semester, do well, start the next semester and drop out. Visits to the emergency room were about to become a pattern, too. Through it all, Alan never stopped looking for real and lasting love.

When Alan was 27, he met a girl named Nicole and seemed to be getting his life back on track. Although Alan didn't get another job, he did go back to school. Nicole spent almost every weekend at our apartment, and the sounds of their conversations and their laughter—even of their arguments—gave me hope. He often romanced Nicki with his poetry. He once wrote to her:

"There aren't enough stars in the sky to account for every time you make me smile."

He frequently told her—as he told all his friends:

"Choose your friends wisely; there are so few you can trust in this world and, ultimately, the only person you can truly trust is yourself."

But loving Nicki presented Alan with a dilemma. As much as he loved and wanted to be with her, there was a secret part of him that warred with that.

When Alan was 15, he'd met a young man from Missouri online. From then until the very moment Alan died, Brandon and Alan would talk on the phone almost daily, even more than once a day. Eventually, Brandon started to talk about the difficulty he was having because he had told his parents that he was gay. Brandon's mother was very religious and totally opposed to this lifestyle. Alan was able to offer advice but, most importantly, he offered unconditional love and support.

When Alan was about 25, he visited Brandon in St. Louis and decided that he was going to move there. I reminded him that a major move might not be a cure for his problems. Later, he sat next to me on the couch and said he had to tell me something. He told me that he was bisexual and in love with Brandon. I hugged him saying:

"All I want is for you to be happy and if Brandon makes you happy, go for it."

He showed me Brandon's picture and had me speak to him on the phone. Alan made a second trip to St. Louis and returned home less eager to relocate. Something had made him see that no matter where he went, he would take his demons with him.

Now, Alan's happiness was marred by his being torn between his love for Nicki and his love for Brandon. He started seeing an LGBT counselor who seemed to be helping him. By reminding Alan that he had been a victim, the counselor helped Alan increase his understanding of many of his problems. Then the counselor moved his practice about 50 miles east of where we lived, and Alan was no longer to get any kind of therapy. Our oppositional relationship began to get even worse.

Life with Alan was clearly not easy but I never for a single moment stopped loving him; never stopped hoping for a better tomorrow. Our relationship was always contentious. I was high-strung and emotional. Alan was stubborn and argumentative. A flammable combination at best and an explosive one at worst.

When Alan was a little boy, I would argue, cajole, and threaten to get him to do what he was supposed to do. As his demons took greater and greater control of him, I would beg him to get out of bed, to go outside, to get exercise. We would argue about his eating habits and the weight he was gaining. He would slam the door to his bedroom. On two occasions, his anger was so great that he punched holes in the bedroom door.

I would remind him constantly – becoming the nag I swore I'd never be – that he was spending more money than I could afford. For a while, he was spending about $1,000 a month to buy Kratom, an herbal supplement that he insisted relieved the back pain he'd been experiencing for a couple of years. Month after month, I borrowed money to pay bills.

At the root of our arguments about money was Alan's deep hatred of being dependent on me and on his knowledge – and guilt – that my supporting him was a serious financial problem. Even though I understood this, it was impossible for me not to lose my temper when he bullied me. In addition, I was terrified that he'd end up homeless after I was gone.

In desperation, I started seeing a psychologist to help me decide if I should practice "tough love" and throw Alan out—something I frequently threatened. Alan came with me to a session and eventually started having his own sessions with this psychologist who believed Alan was too "fragile" to make it out in the world on his own. He believed that my "rejecting" Alan could be a devastating blow.

The psychologist strongly believed that Alan needed to be in an intensive therapeutic program, but none of the programs Alan contacted were accepting new patients. A faster downward spiral was about to begin.

The back pain Alan had been experiencing for years was getting worse, and he was prescribed various opioids. I suspected that all the hours he spent either in bed or hunched over the computer were to blame for the pain, but it turned out that wasn't the case.

Alan finally had an MRI around the fall of 2013 which revealed that he had spina bifida occulta, a condition I never knew existed. I had known about spina bifida which occurs when the spinal cord in a fetus fails to develop or close properly. Spina bifida occulta, the mildest form of this birth defect, is so hidden that it was not detected by amniocentesis when I was pregnant with Alan.

People who have spina bifida occulta may go through their whole life without any symptoms, but some may eventually experience a loss of leg reflexes, leg numbness, and back stiffness. In addition to back pain, the symptoms of spina bifida occulta include depression (apparently *not* a result of the pain) and digestive problems.

Alan certainly suffered from depression *and* had digestive problems. He was always popping antacids and had numerous severe bouts of diarrhea. The general practitioner (GP) who had been seeing Alan for a couple of years thought he had lactose intolerance—one more health professional who didn't connect the dots.

Once Alan knew he had spina bifida occulta, he spent hours on the Internet researching it, but a little knowledge can be a dangerous thing. The information he found opened a door to the darkest and bleakest of futures, and Alan became convinced he would end up in a wheelchair. A horrifying prognosis for any young man, it had to have been excruciating for someone who suffered from lifelong anxiety and depression. In that mental state, he increasingly turned to opioids for relief from pain and to the anti-anxiety and anti-depressant medications he'd been taking for years.

One evening, probably when Alan was 28, Alan was in a remarkably happy mood. We went shopping for a wrench to remove the shower head in his bathroom so that he could put up a detachable hand-held shower head. When we completed our shopping, he suggested we go to eat at his favorite Italian restaurant. He was lively and talkative throughout dinner. When we got home, he seemed a little unsteady on his feet, and then he started to slur his words. I begged him to lie down before he fell down, but he insisted that he was fine.

Alan went into his bedroom and closed the door as usual. I watched TV for a while and then headed to bed, knocking first on his door to kiss him good night. He was clearly stumbling and slurring, and I cautioned him not to take any more meds and to get into bed.

I went to sleep and awakened later to the sound of a persistent rapping. When I went to his door to see what was going on, he was sitting cross-legged on the floor, knocking a small tool against the floor. He looked up at me, but it was clear that he didn't *see* me. He didn't respond when I asked if he was okay. I ran to the phone and dialed 911 to get an ambulance. It was clear Alan had overdosed on one of the many pills the system was filling him with.

Alan was taken out on a stretcher, and, after a number of hours in the emergency room, was admitted to Winthrop University Medical Center. He was furious at being there and argued with everyone who came near him, insisting that he be allowed to go home. A psychiatrist met with him.

Unfortunately, because Alan was an adult and because of medical privacy laws, the psychiatrist was not able to and did not discuss anything with me.

After two days, Alan was discharged with no follow-up plan whatsoever. Is it possible that this type of drug overdose is so common that medical personnel don't think twice about them? Did the medical and psychological professionals at the hospital really think it would be okay to simply send this young man home? Or were they just shrugging their shoulders and dismissing the patient as the special education teachers had dismissed Alan, the student, years before?

For several years, Alan had been seeing a local psychiatrist who continued to prescribe Klonopin for his anxiety along with a variety of antidepressants. None of the drugs seemed to help him emerge from the shadows. Sometimes he recognized that his anxiety and depression were keeping him from being the man he wanted to be, and he would briefly muster the inner resources to do battle.

In November 2012, he posted on Facebook:

To some of you I've been distant. Cold where I used to be warm. Easy to anger. So this is an open letter to those of you I feel I've wronged. I'll always be down. I just let my past utterly suffocate me and I'm sorry for that. I'm going to step up and be the friend, brother, cousin and son and boyfriend that I should have been all along.

And he did try. He started taking classes at NYIT again, got a job, went out of the house more frequently and, of course, tried a different course of drugs.

Over and over, when I insisted he was taking too many pills, Alan would say:

"I know what I'm doing; I'm not stupid."

He certainly wasn't stupid as IQ tests, college grades, and everyone who knew him would attest. Nor was he ignorant. Alan's extensive knowledge of computers, for instance, enabled him to build my computer and several of his own. Having researched every medication he was prescribed, his knowledge of medications was encyclopedic. He quoted Bertrand Russell.

No, he wasn't at all stupid, but his desperate need to escape his physical and emotional pain obliterated all he knew. It was as if his pain was in the driver's seat with his knowledge and his intelligence trapped in the trunk.

Because Alan was over the age of 18, my hands were tied in several ways thanks to a federal law meant to *protect* people. The Health Insurance Portability and Accountability Act, known as HIPAA, is a 1996 federal law that restricts access to individuals' private medical information. Once a person turns 18, even parents cannot access that information.

It was horribly frustrating to be left out of conversations and to be kept in the dark about causes, treatments, and especially prognosis. Alan's mental health care providers wouldn't even talk to me. One actually apologized, saying he knew that I was paying the bills but couldn't give me any information unless Alan gave him permission, which Alan wouldn't do. Alan might have felt that this was at least one way he could assert his independence from me.

I believe that Alan's need to be independent from me clawed at him constantly. He desperately wanted to be his own person, and in charge of his life. These are normal feelings for any young adult, but in Alan's case they were exacerbated by his lack of self-esteem and lifelong feeling that he was different. And, with his intelligence and intuition, he may have had an unconscious realization that the drugs were participating in his loss of independence.

If I wanted access to information without Alan's permission, I would have to go to court to have him declared incapacitated or incompetent. What could possibly be more damaging to Alan's self-esteem than one of these legal pronouncements? I couldn't bear the thought of adding yet another label to those that had already scarred him.

Furthermore, the mountains of paperwork and legal fees seemed to present an insurmountable barrier. I was caught between two terrible choices, and I chose neither.

Now, I feel shame, regret, and guilt, because the damage from the "incompetent" label would have been preferable to a fatal overdose.

A year or so passed and, once again, I found Alan stumbling and slurring. Again, I begged him to get into bed and to not take any more meds. As always he replied with:

"I'm not stupid."

Again, I went to sleep only to be awakened by an odd noise. This time, it sounded almost like tinkling glass. When I went into his room, Alan was sitting on the floor holding the pole of a torchiere lamp and rocking the pole back and forth. One of the glass globes had broken, and the noise was being made when the remaining piece of the globe hit the pole.

This time, Alan didn't even lift his head when I approached. I had to pry the lamp pole out of his hands; he just kept rocking back and forth. Again, I called an ambulance. When I got to the hospital, I sat outside what I guess was a critical-care emergency room. I could hear the nurse saying:

"Breathe, Alan, breathe."

No moment in my life had ever been more terrifying.

I finally got permission to go in and sit next to Alan and hold his hand. An aid had been assigned to stay by his bed to make sure he didn't stop breathing. When his breathing did stabilize, he was moved into the general emergency room area. He was conscious and talking, but he wasn't making any sense.

The psychiatrist who examined Alan almost immediately berated me for being an enabler. How could anyone—a professional or not—pass judgement so quickly? Given that HIPAA prevented my having any input in my son's medical outcomes once he turned 18, how could I be expected to control any of his behaviors?

Then, a social worker arrived and called me aside to discuss treatment options. I was overjoyed, filled with hope that something would finally be done to help my baby. Only now that Alan was non compos mentis was I permitted to discuss his problems with a mental health professional. Now, given Alan's condition, the professionals felt it was in Alan's best interest to get me involved, a determination HIPAA clearly allowed.

The social worker and I had a rather lengthy conversation. I explained to her that Alan had an almost lifelong history of treatment for anxiety and depression, and his current psychologist had urged him to get into an intensive psychiatric program. Alan, too, knew that he was in trouble and had come to believe that an intensive psychological treatment program was his best option.

Having decided that an intensive day program was his best option, Alan would accept nothing less. He had spent many hours online, researching therapists and programs. None of the programs he contacted had openings for new patients but he had been told that he might get a place if he got a referral.

In that moment, having the discussion with the social worker, I thought my prayers had been answered. I thought the social worker's intervention would help Alan secure placement in an intensive program. For a moment, that social worker appeared to be holding a life-preserver that she was prepared to toss my way.

The social worker agreed that Alan's drug use was secondary to his psychological problems and that a drug treatment program would not be appropriate, especially since he wouldn't go to such a program. For the first time in years, I actually saw light at the end of the tunnel.

What happened?

The social worker had Alan placed in a drug treatment program; the very program that she had agreed would not be appropriate. His appointment at the Mineola Treatment Center was scheduled for 12:30 P.M. on December 18th, 2014.

Alan had been sent to this particular facility when he was in high school after having tested positive for marijuana three times during the school's regular drug screenings. His father and I had also been required to go to the center for parent meetings. Parents in the group talked about their children stealing from them and from others. Some even spoke of children who attacked them. Alan had never done anything like that. The program seemed totally wrong for all of us. We all, however, faithfully attended for as long as was required.

Alan's problems since high school had spiraled downward into a deeper, darker place, so it wasn't surprising that Alan was convinced that this same treatment center would not offer the help he now needed. In spite of this conviction, and with much coaxing from both his girlfriend Nicole and me, Alan did keep his initial appointment at the center, but he rejected a repeat of the previous outpatient marijuana treatment protocol.

Alan asked the receptionist at the treatment center for the social worker's contact information so that he could discuss other treatment options with her. The woman from the treatment center who gave him the number mistakenly gave him the social worker's private cell number. When Alan called, the social worker was rather angry and said she'd call back when she was in her office. She never called. The light at the end of the tunnel switched off.

Why did the social worker place Alan in a program *she* had agreed would be inappropriate? Had she even tried to get him placed in an intensive mental health program as we had discussed? Why didn't she return Alan's call after Alan left the treatment center?

Some time after Alan's death, I tried to speak to someone at the hospital to get answers to these questions but to no avail. Eventually, I received a letter from the patient coordinator saying that the psychiatry department had done everything correctly. I wrote back, saying that I considered the social worker had been gravely remiss. No one ever responded.

Each day, I have to wonder whether Alan could have been saved if someone more thorough or responsive or thoughtful had been the social worker. Sometimes I wonder if the cracks in the mental health system had swallowed the social worker, leaving her apathetic or sloppy? And, each day, I wonder if there was something more I could have done.

And so life went on much as it had. Alan's "issues" continued to cause him great physical and emotional pain, but that pain conditioned him to be protective and empathetic when one of his friends was suffering. It is not, then, at all surprising that when Marquand had to move suddenly to accommodate his roommate's aunt, Alan asked if Marquand could temporarily live with us.

From the time Alan and Marquand had met in high school, their friendship had endured even when other friendships had begun to wobble. Other friends Alan had for years became involved in jobs and careers. Some had gotten married. Commonality was lost. One of Alan's closest friends had even turned away when Alan revealed he was bisexual. Marquand, like Alan, was still fighting the demons of anxiety and depression; he and Alan understood and cared for each other as no one else could.

Although I wasn't keen on Marquand's moving in, Alan insisted and—as always—wore me down. How could I say "no" to sheltering someone in the middle of a bitter cold spell? In November 2014, Marquand came to live with us "temporarily." But that temporary arrangement stretched out. Christmas came and Marquand celebrated in my apartment with Nicole and Alan. Then, it was New Year's Eve, and they were all together again. I went to New Jersey to celebrate the holiday with my sister. On the morning of January 1, 2015, Alan and I texted New Year's greetings and our love for each other.

When I got back from my sister's, Alan was looking forward to celebrating his upcoming third anniversary with Nicole on January 11th despite suffering from intense back pain. A few days before New Year's Eve, Alan had visited his general practitioner, and the pain was so bad that Marquand had to help Alan out of the car — a black Nissan that was Alan's pride and joy.

This doctor prescribed gabapentin, a medication that is typically used to treat seizures and the pain associated with shingles. Physicians had also begun to prescribe gabapentin as an alternative to opioids for pain relief. The doctor assured Alan that the gabapentin was totally safe. In retrospect, it appears that was not the case. In April of 2018, CBS news reported that gabapentin had been taken by approximately one-third of those who died from fatal overdoses in Kentucky in 2016.[22] That same report noted that gabapentin could induce blackouts and increase the risk for overdoses. Had the "professionals" failed again?

When Alan and Marquand tried to go out the next day after the trip to the doctor, they discovered that Alan's car would not go into reverse. This was the third time that the transmission had failed. Alan was angry and frustrated and, I think, scared. He knew how tight money was and how upset I'd be. The car was more than ten years old, and it didn't seem practical to replace the transmission again.

When I came home that evening, Alan met me at the door and gave me a big hug.

"What's wrong?" I asked, since he tended to become affectionate when he was troubled.

"Something really good happened," he said.

He had spoken to a very dear friend with whom he'd lost touch, and they'd made arrangements to double date that weekend. Alan was also looking forward to shopping for an anniversary gift for Nicole. He'd asked me to help him decide what to buy, and we'd agreed on a bracelet. Our shopping trip was scheduled for the next day, January 10th. I went to bed that night while Alan and Marquand scoured the Internet for car bargains. When I was trying to fall asleep, Alan came into my bedroom to discuss car choices.

I said, *"Can't you just let me sleep?"*

As always, Alan and Marquand were asleep when I got up on the morning of the 10th, so I headed out to run my errands. They were still sleeping when I returned in the early afternoon. I hated to wake Alan. He got so little sleep and was often very nasty if I did wake him. Several hours passed as I sat in front of the computer, reading email and Facebook posts.

Finally, I decided that I had better wake him so that we could get to the store. Just then, Nicole called to say that she was on her way to the Mineola train station where Alan would have to pick her up. Now it would be difficult if not impossible to get the shopping done before Nicole arrived.

I hurried to knock on Alan's bedroom door; no answer.

I knocked again, louder. Still no answer. Slowly, I opened the door a crack and called:

"Alan, Alan. Get up."

There was no response, so I repeated myself. At that point, Marquand reached up from his mattress on the floor to shake Alan.

"Should he be this cold?" Marquand asked.

I rushed into the room, touched Alan's head, felt the unnatural cold, and ran to call 911.

As I waited for the ambulance, I took the cellphone out of Alan's grasp and clutched his hands. Did I think that if I held on tight enough my baby wouldn't leave? I even opened one of his eyes—how desperately I wanted to see some sign of life.

When the EMTs arrived, they asked me to leave the room, but I heard someone say "coded" and knew that Alan was gone.

All I can remember is sitting on the living room floor, rocking, crying, thinking:

"This time, you didn't make any noise; this time I couldn't save you."

Marquand, too, suffers from guilt:

I was there with Alan at the end and couldn't save him. I'll never get over that. I wish I could've saved you, man, the way you saved me so many times. I hope you're at peace and happy where you are. I'll miss you till my last breath. I love you so much and I feel so alone without you. I can't stop crying, man.

As Marquand lay sleeping on the floor and as I wasted time on the Internet, Alan left us, overdosed on a combination of opioids and benzodiazepines, according to the autopsy report.

"Can't you just let me sleep?" would become the last words I ever said to my baby. Five words that I can't ever erase from my memory.

But, there was life outside that bedroom, demanding that things be done.

I don't remember what I said when I called Erik. I only remember him saying he was on his way from Atlanta.

I called my sister in South Jersey and said:

"Alan's gone."

She asked, *"Gone? Gone where?"*

And then she, too, said she was on her way.

I also had to call a friend to ask if she'd pick Nicki up at the railroad. Poor Nicki knew something wasn't right, but when she came into the apartment, the news totally overwhelmed her.

And so you may think Alan's story ends. But it doesn't, and it won't. The legacy of love that Alan left for me and his brother and father, for Brandon and Nicole, for Marquand, for his aunt and cousins will perpetuate his story. Erik's eulogy for Alan says it better than I ever can:

I am Alan Jacobs' older brother. As many of you probably know, Alan set me up as quite a role model. Now I have to spend the rest of my life trying to live up to the man Alan says I was. To start, I'll make a feeble attempt at remembering him that in no way can capture his wonder. I have three quotes, all related to Alan's life and passions.

First: music

Alan played guitar and bass. He loved music, song, and singing along. There are many anecdotes and stories about Alan's love for music. And there is a quote: "All I know is that I don't know nothing"-from a song called "Knowledge" by Operation Ivy. We all come into this world and are all born knowing nothing. But Alan, in spite of a lack of success with formal schooling, had a thirst for knowledge and drank of the world. Ignorance was probably one of his greatest enemies. Alan was truly brilliant, and was smarter than so many. Alan had a mastery of so many subjects: chemistry, physics, astronomy, philosophy, history, technology, and so on. In losing Alan, we have lost a true Renaissance man.

Know nothing? Alan was the exact opposite, and we all know it. And he challenged us to know more and made us better for it.

Next: Alan loved cars, and also cheesy humor. There are many stories of his jokes or of spending time just riding around with his friends in his many cars through the years.

The remake of the movie Gone in Sixty Seconds had an abundance of both cars and cheesy humor. In the movie, there was a character, Sphinx. For almost the entirety of the movie, Sphinx didn't speak. He was an ogre of a man, a meathead, and you expected him to be nothing more than hired muscle. But, in the end, he proved that you can't judge a book by its cover.

At the very end of the movie, after never saying a word, Sphinx says of a fallen friend:

"If his premature demise has in some way enlightened the rest of you to the grim finish below the glossy veneer of criminal life and inspired you to change your ways, then his death carries with it an inherent nobility. And a supreme glory. We should all be so fortunate. You can say 'Poor Toby.' I say: 'Poor us.'"

To so many in this room, Alan was confidant, counselor, adviser, trusted companion, and true friend. The Facebook outpouring showed what a true difference he made in so many lives. In so many ways, Alan's own experiences helped him help others. They helped him understand what others were going through. They helped him talk others off ledges he himself had looked out from. I don't wish his experiences on anyone, but in a way, we are better off for his carrying them.

So many have said that Alan was always there at the drop of a hat to help, to console, and to comfort, at any hour. Many may look at his life and say "poor Alan." I say "poor us." The world is forever lighter, and our hearts forever heavier for his loss.

Finally, philosophy. It is clear that he loved it from the kind words shared by Dr. Navia [Alan's philosophy professor who also spoke at the funeral]. A Scottish poet, Thomas Campbell (1777-1844) said:

"To live in hearts we leave behind is not to die."

A good friend who had suffered from personal demons for much of her life posted that on my Facebook page, and it is so true. There are so many photos of Alan's smile - a smile that bore his soul for the world to see and enjoy. If you were lucky enough to know it, or his laugh, you had received a true gift.

We are so fortunate to have the technology that we do. At Walgreens last night, we printed these photos of Alan, and we realized: Push a button, and Alan is there. On Facebook, in your phones, in your photo albums, and on YouTube, Alan will always be there for us with the swipe of a finger, at the click of a mouse. He may be gone from our physical world, but we can still talk to him, and still get advice from him, and call on him at any moment, simply by calling on each other and on his memory. Alan still lives on in all of us and we are all more closely connected than at any time in history. Through us and our connections, we keep Alan alive for eternity, until we meet again.

Finally, I call on you: Know something. Especially one another.

Feel sorry not for Alan, but for us. For losing someone so great.

Keep him alive through your memory and your relationships.

And, ultimately, do not let his torch dim, for through his, we not only light our own, but grow brighter and burn longer for it.

To Alan. Rest in peace. I hope you found what you were looking for. I think about you almost every day. I hope you know that as proud as you are of me, I am so much prouder of you, for being stronger in so many ways than I ever could or will be.

Erik's moving words go far in capturing the essence of Alan, who was more—so much more — than his mental health issues, more than his dependence on pills, more than the words on these pages.

This book is my way of passing Alan's torch on to others. Our reading and sharing the words here is one way to keep that torch burning. The friends whose lives Alan so deeply touched is another: the love he showed them, the lessons he imparted live on.

Alan's friend Kenneth is just one example. He and Alan had been very close since their teen years but had a falling out about a year before Alan's death. Ken was devastated that they hadn't had the time to make things right. In remembering Alan, he said

It's absolutely astonishing how much love he gave all the while he was screaming inside. The only time I have ever known Alan to fail in love was in finding the love he owed to himself.

Ken's post on Facebook is a poignant testimony to Alan's devotion to his friends:

Today I lost my best friend.... he was the only proof I've ever known that angels might exist. I love you Alan Jacobs. You gave me a part of yourself that will forever live in my heart. In the wake of loss, the best you can do is try to make sense of it. I will always love and miss you, Alan .....

if you were here, you'd be pushing me in the direction of my passions and dreams... I'll catch you on the flip side of things, buddy. Until then I'll just have to live for the both of us.

Alan's friendships were so deep and true that I have been blessed by the continuing presence in my life of Ken, Marquand, and Adrianna.

I thank Alan for that gift and for the important lesson he taught us: Fear is the greatest enemy we have: fear of shame and stigma, fear of the unknown keeps too many of us silent when we should be bringing those fears out into the open.

Fears grow and fester and rot in the darkness, eventually obscuring the light, robbing the chance of joy, of life.

PTSD

"The rockets' red glare, the bombs bursting in air…" The words of our national anthem are meant to remind us of the bravery of those who fought to defend our freedom. For some, the words also stir memories of weapons of warfare and the devastation they bring. Exploding shells ravage the landscape and rip limbs, sight, hearing and life from soldiers. Sometimes the effects of the blasts leave wounds that maim the mind rather than the body. Less than a year after the beginning of World War I, battlefield soldiers began to exhibit severe trembling, dizziness, confusion, loss of memory and sleep disorders. These were attributed to "the severe concussive motion of the shaken brain in the soldier's skull."[23]

The phenomenon came to be known as "shell shock." Initially removed to peaceful surroundings far from the battle front, those with shell shock were later treated at the front lines. Subsequently, shell shocked soldiers were treated at the front lines with rest, psychotherapy and, sometimes, hydrotherapy or electrotherapy, with the hope of returning the soldiers to battle as quickly as possible.

World War I came to an end, but it would not be the "war to end all wars." A scant two decades later, the world became engulfed in World War II.

Building on the thoughts from World War I, an attempt was made to screen draftees for eligibility based on whether or not the draftee might be resilient under pressure. The effort failed. "Of the 800,000 American troops who actually saw combat during the Second World War, 37.5 percent displayed such severe psychological symptoms that they were permanently discharged."[24]

Then came the Vietnam War, and "an estimated 700,000 Vietnam veterans - almost a quarter of all soldiers sent to Vietnam from 1964 to 1973 - required some form of psychological help."[25]

In 1980, the American Psychiatric Association included post traumatic stress disorder (PTSD) in its diagnostic "Bible," *The Diagnostic and Statistical Manual of Mental Disorders* (DSM-lll), for the first time. According to Matthew J. Friedman, M.D., Ph.D., "…the significant change ushered in by the PTSD concept was the stipulation that the etiological agent was outside the individual (i.e., a traumatic event) rather than an inherent individual weakness (i.e., a traumatic neurosis)."[26] "Post traumatic stress disorder" would soon be known to everyone.

According to the Diagnostic Manual, there are more than a dozen symptoms of PTSD, a number of which must be present for at least one month for the diagnosis of PTSD to be given. Alan exhibited at least eight of the symptoms, including:

- recurrent distressing dreams of the event
- efforts to avoid thoughts or feelings associated with the trauma
- efforts to avoid activities or situations that arouse recollections of the trauma
- inability to recall an important aspect of the trauma (psychogenic amnesia)
- in young children, loss of recently acquired developmental skills such as toilet training or language skills
- difficulty falling or staying asleep
- irritability or outbursts of anger
- difficulty concentrating

War veterans aren't the only ones who experience PTSD: it is estimated that 24.4 million Americans have PTSD as a result of such events as abuse, accidents, and disasters. The National Institute of Health defines PTSD as "a disorder that develops in some people who have experienced a shocking, scary, or dangerous event."[27] Some of these people also experience PTSD because of the sudden death of a loved one or when a family member experiences harm or danger.[28]

Alan was born in 1986, six years after the publication of the DSM-III which introduced PTSD as a diagnosis. By the time Alan's problems arose, PTSD should have been well known by mental health professionals. How is it possible that the mental health professionals seemed unable or unwilling to consider that Alan might have had issues beyond or even other than ADHD?

Because he was repressing memories (experiencing psychogenic amnesia), the truth about his sexual abuse didn't come out until Alan was about 18. Even without this piece of the puzzle, it should have been obvious that he'd experienced "shocking, scary, or dangerous events" such as his maternal grandmother's loss of vision, his paternal grandmother's death, and his father's life-threatening medical issues.

Did they skip over PTSD because in the mid 80s a diagnosis of ADHD was almost a foregone conclusion for any child — especially a boy — who acted out and didn't neatly fit into a school system's idea of an ideal student?

This trend of applying the ADHD diagnosis to all children has not abated. In reality, the number of children diagnosed keeps increasing —7.8 percent in 2003 to 9.5 percent in 2007 to 11 percent in 2016.[29] But the number of children suffering from PTSD is barely recognized. A British study of more than 2000 18-year-olds reported in 2019 that "almost one in 13 (8%) suffer from PTSD following a childhood trauma. …Among those with PTSD, only one in five had ever received any professional help."[30]

Through the years, I pointed out to many mental health professionals that Alan's problems all seemed to start at a rather specific time. Before he started school, he had been the "best boy." Once in school, he became angry and defiant and started to wet the bed at night. Not a single professional ever seemed to consider that a sudden onset of symptoms could have been related to a trauma or that there was a possibility of post-traumatic stress disorder.

Hopefully, this lack of awareness will change now that a comprehensive review of more than 230,000 adults has revealed that sexual assault is "associated with increased risk for all forms of psychopathology assessed, and relatively stronger associations were observed for posttraumatic stress and suicidality."[31]

My feeling that psychologists and psychiatrists failed Alan by not recognizing his PTSD symptoms haunts me almost every single day. How could the professionals have missed that diagnosis? Were they trained adequately — or at all — in the symptoms and treatment of PTSD? When major changes to the DSM are introduced, how does the psychological community ensure that its professionals stay up to date? Did Alan just present those symptoms too long before anyone other than a soldier received that diagnosis?

It now seems to me that Alan's resumption of bed-wetting was a significant symptom indicative of PTSD. When I think about the pages and pages of reports about Alan and all the labels in them, the following lines constantly jolt—and anger —me:

"No history of head trauma, motor vehicle accidents, lost consciousness or seizures. ... Attained bladder and bowel control at age three. About a year later, Alan started to wet the bed and stopped at around age nine."

Why is the list of possible traumas limited to those with clear physio-neurological implications? Why did no one delve into the mystery of resumption of bed-wetting, which—even without considering PTSD —is often caused by psychological stress? Didn't any of the psychologists know that "Often bedwetting can be seen as an unconscious signal that home is not a safe place to be. For children, this can include divorce, abuse, or neglect, and even a response to alcoholism in the family."[32] The National Institute of Mental Health points out that in children under 6, resumption of bed-wetting after having been trained can be a symptom of PTSD.[33]

Once again, signs that Alan had experienced a trauma around the time he started school should have been clear to the mental health professionals. How could the signs have been ignored? If there had been an Internet then, perhaps my access to information would have motivated me to convince the professionals to actually consider that a trauma had caused many—if not all—of his problems.

Partly because I was sure Alan's trauma had to do with the harm his loved ones had experienced (the various medical issues and deaths in the close family) and partly because I was totally naïve about his sexual abuse, I had missed an important sign. I didn't even know it was a sign until I started doing research for this book and learned that one of the symptoms associated with PTSD is "acting out the scary event during playtime."[33]

When Alan was in first grade, I often walked him into class. One morning, the teacher asked if she could have a word with me. When we stepped outside the door, she told me quietly and politely that Alan had exposed himself in the school yard the day before. I was horrified and mortified. I asked to have a word with Alan, and we walked to an empty spot near the school entrance. There were no tears and no yelling, but I definitely came down hard, telling him how shameful his action was and warning him to never ever repeat it.

If I had only known that exposing himself might have indicated he'd experienced sexual abuse, he might have gotten the appropriate psychological guidance right from the start. Can I really lay blame at the feet of the mental health professionals when I saw and suspected nothing? Should a mother have understood her child even better than the professionals did? Is it necessary for parents and educators to be versed in the intricacies of psychoanalysis?

Perhaps everyone in Alan's life would have acted differently if these events were happening today. Although it is very likely that pedophiles and sex abusers have been living among us for millennia, only in the last two decades has the public really become conscious and aware of them due to the heightened media attention on sex abuse scandals involving priests, Coach Jerry Sandusky at Penn State, Larry Nassar and the USA Gymnastics scandal, and, unfortunately and sadly, countless others.

Hopefully today, parents, school personnel and mental health professionals are more likely to investigate the possibility of sexual abuse when youngsters display certain behavioral problems.

PART TWO

Death, be not proud, though some have called thee
Mighty and dreadful, for thou are not so;
For those whom thou think'st thou dost overthrow
Die not, poor Death…
From "Death, be not proud"

By John Donne

A Broken Heart

The names of all the people at Brunswick Hospital have been changed.

How do I find words to express what I felt after Alan died? I can't.

Shock after great trauma protects the mind, and, for the first month or so, the shock allowed me to be totally disconnected from the awful reality. I walked around in a haze although I cried every morning when I woke up and every time I saw a picture of Alan. Pictures that weren't hanging on walls were turned over, waiting for the day when I could look at them.

The first weeks were a flurry of people and activity. Erik came from Atlanta, Georgia, along with his wife, as soon as he heard the news. My sister, Tema, came from New Jersey as quickly as traffic would allow. They were followed shortly by my niece and nephew and their families. And Marquand was ever present.

Erik, Ainsley, my sister and I made the funeral arrangements although Erik and Ainsley really did most of it, getting Alan's clothes ready, picking out the pictures for the funeral and even paying the horrific sum of $12,000 for the casket and funeral services.

Alan would be buried with my parents—the grandpa he never knew but so resembled and his beloved Gram'Bea — in a plot in New Jersey with his Uncle Roger—my sister's husband — close by. In my mind, I could see them welcoming him as he crossed over.

The funeral actually brought me some measure of comfort. I was amazed by the number of people who came to the funeral service. So many of Alan's friends—past and present—some known to me, others complete strangers, attended. It was standing room only, just as my father's funeral had been more than 50 years before. Like my father, Alan had touched every life he came in contact with.

Time and again as Alan's friends came up to offer condolences, they mentioned how he had helped them through tough times. Having lived with his own demons for so long, Alan knew the words needed to talk to others' demons. Sadly, Alan could never find the strength to confront his own demons.

I managed — with the help of a Xanax — to find the strength to speak at the funeral. As I recall I asked Alan's friends — or begged them — to remember him by living the lives he'd told them they could have.

On the way to the New Jersey cemetery from the funeral home in Queens, numbness took over. Everyone in the car chatted, but I cannot recall a word or even a topic. We were greeted at the cemetery by a rabbi who I had never previously met. He was hired by the funeral home to say the appropriate prayer at the grave.

As the rabbi was asking people to throw a spade of dirt into the grave, I walked away, back to the waiting limousine. It was impossible— heartrending beyond belief—to watch them put my baby under the earth. I can't write this without crying. I can't ever think of Alan in his grave. That is a horror I do not have the strength to confront and suspect I never will.

When we finally arrived home from the funeral activities, I found my apartment filled with the friends who had most loved and been closest to Alan. Several asked for mementoes to remember him by. Later, Erik, Ainsley, and Marquand got down to cleaning out the detritus of a lifetime of unfinished plans, dreams, and projects. Every now and then, I'd watch from the bedroom door. There were no tears. Instead I felt relieved at finally getting rid of the horrid mess:

The microphones, amps, music books, and guitars from his desire to be a rock musician.

The apron, gloves, and tools from when he decided to become a blacksmith.

Boxes of ammunition and gun cleaning equipment from his target-shooting days.

Hard drives, flash drives, tools, books, and scores of cables from his information technology career.

Two axes, the purpose of which I can no longer recall.

And his books — mostly Terry Pratchett's *Discworld* series — every one of which he had read over and over.

In another age, with a patron or wealthy parents, Alan would have been revered as a Renaissance man.

My cupboards and refrigerator were cleaned out, too. It was impossible to eat—or even look at —any of Alan's favorite foods. Feeding Alan had been my way of expressing my love and concern. So much else seemed to end up reduced to nagging. For months after his death, I couldn't go to a supermarket without crying, and cooking became an insurmountable feat. I lived on frozen prepared foods and ramen noodles. The psychologist had urged me to be good to myself, so I indulged in a lot of candy and fast food.

During those first few weeks, posts on Alan's Facebook page came quickly and were heartfelt. One friend even created a YouTube video comprised of a collage of pictures of Alan (http://bit.ly/alan-youtube-collage). Watching that video, seeing Alan smiling and joking with his friends, warmed my heart. It reminded me that Alan's life hadn't always been one of misery and anxiety.

All too soon, though, Erik and Ainsley and my niece and nephew returned to their lives in Georgia and Virginia. About a week after the funeral, my sister also returned to her life, which included a much anticipated and long-planned trip to India.

Each morning, I woke and started crying, which was invariably followed by panic attacks—how odd when the worst had already happened. Sometimes all I could feel was horror. Sometimes I raged and threw things.

Marquand was still living with me, but, despite his presence, I was alone.

In that loneliness, I was plagued by guilt. All the should-haves and could-haves ran through my head on constant replay:

A mother's first job is to protect her children, and I had failed at that.

I spent too much time away from Alan.

I didn't absolutely insist that he eat dinner at the table with me.

I didn't educate myself enough about mental health.

I was 66 and alive. My son, not yet 30, was dead. Parents shouldn't outlive their children.

I didn't fight the professionals hard enough.

Why didn't my conviction that Alan had suffered a trauma spur me to fight harder?

Throughout Alan's life, I had always connected the trauma to the death of Alan's grandmother and his father's sickness coming so close together. Never did the possibility of sexual abuse enter my mind. Why would it have? My boys had been told that no one could touch the parts of their bodies that their swimming trunks covered. They were never left in the care of strangers. I was naïve.

Somehow, I managed to keep putting one foot in front of the other and kept going despite the grief and guilt and pain. I went back to work, watched TV, read books, and even met my friends for dinners. Life resumed a pattern that in my better moments I referred to as the "new normal." In other moments, when the silence surrounded me, I often thought of just how "not normal" Alan's loss was.

Death is, after all, part of the cycle of life, but the death of a loved one is always painful. When a parent dies, the age of the child profoundly affects the nature of the loss. One thing is always true: Loss of a parent is loss of a constant, loss of the one truly unconditional love there is. When a beloved spouse passes, we lose a friend, a lover, a partner. We may feel we've lost an anchor. When a sibling dies, we lose a playmate, a confidante, a companion. No one can ever provide that link to our history. There is an empty space in our life experience.

When we lose a child, we lose a piece of ourselves—our blood ran through those veins. Our hopes and dreams disappear. And there is a sense of horror: The death of a child is so wrong that the universe spins into chaos—there are no rules, no order. Parents are supposed to die first; parents are not supposed to bury their children. Children should not die while aging parents walk on.

Human beings find it very difficult to grapple with the idea that the universe might be completely random, or that things don't always happen for a reason. All our lives, we're trained to think in terms of consequences.

We need reasons why tragedy strikes even the best among us. A young man with a brilliant mind, a quick wit, and a heart more caring than most is plagued by a myriad of events in his past, fears for his future, and physical pain. He takes his prescription pills and then takes just one—or two, or even three—more to relieve the pain and fear and memory. We ask, "Why him?" That way madness lies. There are no answers. The best we can do is be in the moment.

When my planned or required activities were done, there was nothing for me but the pain of missing Alan and the feeling that I had totally failed as a mother. My hunger to be with him never left me, nor did my belief that it should have been me that had died. Whenever I got in my car, I'd start to cry again. All I wanted was Alan. I started to think that if I was dead, I'd be with him again.

After my father died, an old friend of my mother's had said that all of our dead relatives would be lined up to welcome us when we died. I found myself often remembering her statement. And then I kept remembering—even hearing—Natalie Wood in the original *Miracle on 34th Street*. She had lost her belief in Santa Claus when Santa hadn't gotten her the house she longed for. Leaving a Christmas party, little Natalie sat in the back of the car repeating, *"I believe. I believe."* I kept repeating it to myself, too. *"I believe I can be with Alan again."*

And so, I started planning my journey.

I wrote in my journal, *"I believe that I will be with my son again one day. Right now I don't intend to wait long either. I know that Erik and Tema will be heart-broken, but I've always believed that each of us ultimately has the choice of living or dying. This time, I'll be selfish. I'll choose the path that I believe is best for me. It's not that I can't stand it, but that I refuse to do so.*" A suicide attempt was, at least in part, a way to seize control from the chaos.

My physician had prescribed Xanax for me to help me deal with the anxiety and stress that living with Alan's problems had been causing. I still had two bottles that I hadn't taken, and I was able to get a new prescription because the doctor didn't know I still had so many pills left. Now, I had three bottles. Would that be enough?

I read online about various drugs, searching for the ones that could lead to respiratory failure and death. I also had vodka that I was going to drink when I took the pills. My only fears were that I'd vomit before the pills could take effect —so I took an antiemetic that would prevent that. The possibility that I'd end up in a vegetative state also frightened me: if I cared about anything real at that time it was that I not be a burden to Erik.

I arranged my finances and cleaned out a lot of clothing and other belongings, donating them to a veterans' organization and to Big Brothers/Big sisters. CDs were sold, books were donated to Books4Cause, and a list of my computer passwords and a contact list were compiled. Of course, I wrote Erik a letter of explanation. Wanting to spare Marquand from having to find me, too, I made a reservation at a local motel. Ultimately, I decided that I really wanted to lie down in my own bed, with Alan's pictures around me, and snuggle up with the hat that Alan always wore.

At 8 P.M. on the night of April 24th, 2015, I sat down on the couch with my drink and three bottles of Xanax and turned the TV on. I planned to take the first bottle of pills with the vodka, take the rest as soon as I started to feel sleepy, and then head to bed. Little did I know that one bottle of pills and the vodka would so quickly render me unconscious.

At some point that night—maybe about 11 P.M.—Marquand came home and found me sleeping on the couch. He covered me and went into his room. When he came out, an hour or so later, I was still sleeping on the couch. Becoming concerned by my slow and shallow breathing, he sat next to me for a time and then called Alan's father. The decision was made to call 911, and I was rushed to the emergency room at Winthrop University Hospital near my home.

I don't remember anything of the next 24 hours. The first I knew after having taken those pills and that drink, I opened my eyes to see Ken and Marquand standing at the foot of my bed, holding a stuffed cat and flowers. Erik and my niece were standing next to the bed. I realized that my suicide attempt had failed, but I felt nothing—neither disappointment, nor anger, nor joy. Maybe the pills had a residual tranquilizing effect.

In my drug-induced daze, I wondered if Alan had somehow interceded. I don't really believe that happened, but throughout my life I've wondered about the possibility of ghosts. I never really believed they existed, and I've never really believed in an afterlife, either. I think those possibilities became something of a lifeline after Alan died. The possibility that I could be with him in death or that he could come to me as a spirit provided some solace.

After the emergency room, I was in a hospital room for about two days before being transferred to a mental health facility. According to New York State law, an "allegedly mentally ill person" can be committed if close family members or "professionals familiar with the individual's lifestyle and behavior patterns...request or submit an application" for that commitment. "Two physicians must then agree and present documentation that the person has a mental illness necessitating inpatient care and treatment. ... If the hospital has inpatient psychiatric treatment facilities, a third evaluation is performed by a staff psychiatrist to confirm whether or not the individual meets state standards for involuntary commitment."[34]

Presumably all of these steps had been taken although I have no recollection of answering any questions or discussing my mental state with anyone. To this day I can remember almost nothing about my emergency room or hospital stay. If I can't even remember the time I was in the emergency room or in the hospital bed, it doesn't seem possible that I would have been sufficiently compos mentis to answer questions from two different physicians. What criteria were used to determine I was "at risk"? While some statistics say that "8.6% of individuals admitted to a psychiatric unit with suicidal ideation or after a suicide attempt will eventually die by suicide,"[34] was that statistic sufficient evidence for me to be involuntarily committed?

Why was I more at risk than Alan had been after his *second* overdose? Are failed suicide attempts more often repeated than accidental drug overdoses? A psychiatrist and social worker in the *very same* emergency room in the *very same* hospital had thought Alan could be helped simply with counseling and recommended an outpatient treatment program for him. Wouldn't it also have been possible for me to get help as an outpatient?

I would find out later, in passing, that my having made a detailed suicide plan, instead of an impulsive suicide attempt in a moment of intense grief, meant I was seriously depressed.

Oddly, the three and a half months after Alan died hadn't felt like a period of serious depression. Aside from sleeping more than usual, I was living "normally." In fact, my apparently normal lifestyle made it impossible for the psychologist I was seeing regularly, or my family and friends, to think that I was suicidal.

My "depression" certainly wasn't a textbook case. It was not marked by lack of hope, feelings of worthlessness, or a loss of motivation. For many, a suicide attempt and depression both have hopelessness at the core. But hope was the basis of my suicide attempt — the hope that I'd be with my son again.

None of that mattered. A decision was made to commit or lock me up without any discussion with me. If I'd been a criminal, I'd at least have been read my Miranda rights. No one discussed any options with Erik, either. He was thrust into a panicked fit of research, trying to select from a list of state-sponsored and -funded institutions since my finances and insurance wouldn't cover a high-end private facility. In addition, because private institutions are out of the reach of many, the public institutions are usually at capacity and often cannot take new patients. Even if Erik had chosen the very best facility from the list of possibilities, it was possible there would have been no bed for me. This lack of beds is part of the reason that I was kept in the purgatory between the emergency room and the psychiatric hospital for two days. The "powers that be" had committed me to inpatient psychiatric care, but I was not receiving *any* psychiatric care in the regular hospital.

Whether I was truly depressed or not, I was about to discover firsthand just how broken the mental health care system in the U.S. is.

When I was finally discharged from the hospital, I was put on a stretcher to be transported to the psychiatric hospital. I remember thinking *"I hope it's not like* The Snake Pit.*"* This 1948 movie starring Olivia de Havilland had depicted the horrors of the insane asylums that predated psychiatric hospitals. The movie's vivid and frightening images of patients being herded into a hole like animals and of nurses' cruelty to the patients had apparently stayed in my subconscious. In reality, it turned out that I was heading for another version of *One Flew Over the Cuckoo's Nest.*

The ride in the ambulance lasted about half an hour. I watched the passing scenery and could see Erik and Ainsley following the ambulance in my car. When we pulled into the driveway of the Brunswick Hospital Center in Amityville, New York, I was pleasantly surprised. A cinder block building surrounded by a lawn, some trees, and picnic tables came into view.

"Oh, this isn't so bad," I thought.

I was wheeled into the admitting room where I signed some papers and was told it was dinnertime.

"We're known for having good food," said the woman in admitting as my stretcher was wheeled through double doors that had to be unlocked to allow us to enter.

I don't recall the doors slamming with a thud behind me, but they might as well have done so. Ainsley and Erik left the hospital without really being able to see me, but they had instructions to return later during visiting hours with clothing and books for me. My isolation from the real world of home and friends and cat was about to become complete —I was even isolated from my clothing.

I had urinated on my clothes when the overdose rendered me unconscious and had been wearing only a hospital gown during my time at

Winthrop. No one at Winthrop told Erik he could bring clothing for me to wear in the psychiatric hospital. When I arrived at Brunswick, I was given two new hospital gowns to dress in — one to wear in front and one to wear in back. Then I was met by a nurse who had me remove the shoelaces from my sneakers. She then performed a pat down. I'm not sure where I could have been hiding anything in the two hospital gowns that they had given me.

Later I would surmise that this procedure was probably standard because of the number of addicts and psychotics that came into the facility. Women, especially, have extra hiding places for contraband. I wonder if some patients receive even more dehumanizing searches?

The nurse then escorted me into a colorless dining room totally devoid of any decoration. There were windows, but they were covered with wire screens so dense they barely let in any light. Were the screens keeping people outside or keeping us inside? I quickly began to feel like I was being incarcerated rather than institutionalized. Then again, they do call prisons "institutions."

Several round tables were scattered around the room with a total of about 15 people seated at them. Alone and frightened, I kept my eyes down but couldn't help seeing an elderly lady in a wheelchair, and a very disheveled and greasy-haired woman who had a totally unfocused look. There were also several other messy-looking, overweight women in hospital gowns. Seated alone at a corner table was a morbidly obese man wearing a hospital gown, muttering to himself.

For a facility whose purpose was to help individuals deal with their mental health problems, there were an awful lot of dehumanizing hospital gowns.

Conversation at most of the tables was sporadic or non-existent, but at one table a group of three youngish women was chatting loudly and laughing uproariously. They made me think of "mad hatters" or the three witches who open the play *Macbeth* by intoning, "Double, double, toil and trouble/Fire burn, and cauldron bubble." The witches predict the downfall of the main character, and the echo of their ominous foreboding seemed to foretell that my slide into a world of insanity was just beginning.

Through it all, seated by the room's only door was an attendant, keeping a watchful eye on everyone. For a person like me who is nervous, high strung, and fiercely independent, this setting made me feel as if I had, indeed, ended up in *Snakepit.* Having seen the movie when I was an adolescent, the disturbing images had left a deep impression. Maybe the impression that *Snakepit* had left explains why the individuals in the dining room seemed to me to have grotesque characteristics.

Tormented by misgivings, I sat silently and chewed without tasting the slightly cool cheeseburger on the paper plate in front of me. I didn't touch the incredibly limp-looking fries next to the burger. Concentrating on chewing and swallowing, I looked at no one until I felt someone lean close to my ear, quickly place a hand on my shoulder and say,

"Don't worry. It will be okay." That was Amy.

Without her friendship, compassion and humor, I think I might actually have lost my sanity over the next 21 days. She and the other two women sitting with her were not "Mad Hatters" at all, nor did they have any witch-like characteristics. My initial impression that they were "cackling" was, no doubt, fueled by my extreme anxiety at being in a mental hospital.

Two of these young women had attempted suicide and had been committed to the hospital just like me. The third woman had voluntarily committed herself when she realized that she had become dependent on pills after the death of her husband. Incessant chatter and laughter were these women's way of coping with a situation that was, by turns, bizarre, frustrating, humiliating, and once or twice even frightening.

In the laughter and friendship of these women, I found a lifeline.

After dinner, Erik and Ainsley came to visit. Visitors had to be escorted into the dining room, which also served as the visitors' room. Erik brought the stuffed cat that Ken gave me in the hospital to remind me of Koshka, along with some supplies. The guard at the visiting room door— actually a psychiatric aide (PA)—asked him to empty out the bag. For unclear reasons, we were told that I could not keep the stuffed cat. Several hard-covered books were also prohibited. We learned that their size and heft meant they could potentially turn into dangerous weapons, especially if thrown. The drawstrings on my pajama bottoms were removed, as they, like the shoelaces, presented a risk of suicide by strangulation. Lastly, the scrunchie I used to hold my pony tail was also taken away, but for what reason I am still unsure.

Erik had brought my prescription medications, but they, too, were contraband even though I'd been taking them for years. They had been prescribed by my personal physician and were in the prescription pill bottles, clearly labeled by the dispensing pharmacy. Included in that medicine assortment was blood pressure medication.

Fortunately for me, not having my blood pressure medication for a short time would not be fatal. But what about for someone else? The toiletries kit I'd been given at Winthrop contained ear plugs and mouthwash. For some reason, the ear plugs were contraband; the body wash, however, was allowed and was taken away to be put in my personal "bin." This plastic shoe box had my first name on it and was kept in a locked closet opposite the two shared bathrooms — one for men and one for women.

Later that evening, I met with a physician who briefly reviewed my history. After this intake meeting with the medical doctor, I didn't see a physician again — none of the patients did — unless we asked, and asked, and asked again. I didn't see the psychiatrist then because it was a Saturday evening, and the psychiatrist who had been assigned to me wouldn't be in until Sunday.

After the physician's meeting, it was time to get ready for bed. In order for me to get to my toiletries, a member of the staff had to unlock the closet. I was given my bin which contained a toothbrush, the worst-tasting toothpaste on the planet, a comb and a hair brush. When I was finished in the bathroom, the box was returned to the closet, which was locked again.

On a few occasions, there was no one to open the closet when I left the bathroom, so I put the bin on a shelf in my room. Each time I did this, the bin was removed during the night. Obviously this was inconvenient, but it was also dehumanizing, taking away any feeling that my life belonged to me and reminding me constantly that privacy was out of the question.

Bedtime came, and I was shown to my room. There were two beds, and each had a foam mattress with a rubberized covering on a wooden base. There were no drawers in the room. Only open shelves were provided for our clothing. In that way, the staff could easily see if we had food or any other forbidden items in the room. Chapstick or a pen were forbidden. Pencils were allowed. It would appear that stabbing another patient to death with a writing implement would be okay, but bludgeoning them or strangling them would not.

In the room there was also a desk that was bolted to the floor along with a plastic chair. Drab gray-white walls were unadorned except for a chalkboard that each day announced the name of the day nurse and the PA on duty. Little natural light came into the room as the locked windows were covered in the same dense screening used in the dining room. Few members of the staff had keys to these locked windows. If we wanted them opened or closed, a staff member had to go outside the building to do it.

Although there were two beds, I had no roommate the first night. That was a relief, no matter how small. I'd never gone to sleepaway camp or roomed in a dormitory. My sister, my mother, and my husband had been the only roommates I'd ever known. The possibility of rooming with a complete stranger was frightening.

After getting into the bed, I closed my eyes, but sleep was out of the question. The woman in the room next to mine screamed *"Get me out of here"* all night long. Was she being held against her will? Was I? The woman also incessantly called for the nurse, or for water, or to get physical assistance go to the bathroom. In spite of the noise, I wasn't allowed to shut my door.

It seemed barely light outside when there was a pounding on my open door, and a loud voice yelled *"Vitals."* According to the clock in the hallway, it was barely 6 A.M. Patients lined up in the hallway to have their blood pressure and temperature taken. On Mondays, we were also weighed.

Breakfast wouldn't be until 7 A.M., so many of us sat around in the day room to pass the time. The day room, as the name suggests, was where we spent our days, coloring, staring at the TV, chatting, having group meetings.

The day room had a row of bolted-down plastic chairs against one wall. On the opposite wall, there was a TV, a refrigerator, and a table with some moveable chairs around it. At the other end of the room, there were three chairs with plastic-covered upholstery and also bolted to the floor. In the corner was a pay phone, which we were allowed to use for a couple of hours in the morning and a couple of hours in the evening (cell phones were forbidden).

Two walls had windows, but, again, the dense screens prevented the room from ever being really bright. The TV was always on unless there was some sort of group meeting being held in the room. The only way to change the channel or adjust the volume was to find a staff member who then had to get the remote control out of the locked nurse's office. The staff didn't want to risk someone throwing the remote, but apparently the few chairs that weren't bolted down presented an acceptable level of risk. The setting was straight out of *One Flew Over the Cuckoo's Nest.*

If we needed anything, we'd have to knock on the office door and wait to be acknowledged. Many times we would have to shout through the door because the doctor or nurse at the desk couldn't be bothered to get up to open it.

At breakfast on the second day, I sat with the three laughing ladies and started to learn their stories. Although we were in a geriatric ward, my new friends' ages ranged from 20 to 45.

Evie, who was almost 40, had been admitted after a failed suicide attempt. She'd been diagnosed with a spinal tumor. Although the surgery to remove it was successful, it left her with a steel rod in her back. Not only did she deal with constant pain, but she always feared that the tumor would return.

Evie had the kind of beauty that made people turn to look at her. Her long, straight hair was a shiny black, and she had beautiful eyes and an amazing figure. Sadly, most of those who looked at her never got to know her inner beauty — her amazing generosity, love of others, wit and intellectual curiosity.

Another of the young women, Amy, also had attempted suicide. She'd lost a child late in pregnancy and had had several miscarriages. Subsequently, she developed an immune condition that left her too fatigued to work.

The third woman had admitted herself because she'd become addicted to Xanax after the lengthy illness and death of her young husband.

Our group also sometimes included a woman of only 20 who was waiting to be transferred to a drug rehabilitation facility. Apparently Brunswick could serve as both psychiatric hospital and holding area.

Several other patients were also recovering drug addicts, and there were schizophrenics, too. Was commitment to a ward of diagnosed psychotics and drug addicts really helpful to depressed individuals at risk of repeated suicide attempts? I often felt that I would lose my sanity if I had to listen to the screams, cackles, and ramblings of the inmates for one more day.

The "three witches'" ability to laugh at it all and their willingness to listen to me and share their tears and fears with candor and genuine caring made it all bearable — if only just. If they were witches, they were certainly the Good Witches of the East.

The "witches'" sense of humor was infectious. Throughout our hospitalization, we always managed to find humor in our situation as well as in that of the other "inmates," as I started calling them.

In many ways, we were behaving like high school students who were the in-crowd making fun of the nerds and geeks. Certainly it was wrong to make fun of people who were suffering from mental illness, but we so needed to release our fears and frustrations. Although we laughed, we also were always ready to lend a hand when others needed something.

Evie was especially compassionate. She always rushed to help the women who were in wheelchairs, picking up items they dropped or helping them push their chairs when necessary. At snack time, Evie sometimes helped one of the elderly women open the cookie packages or peel an orange. She was the first to run to get a glass of water for an elderly patient who was choking on her pills.

Amy became something of a den mother to the terribly disheveled and shy patient I'd spotted in the dining room. Amy engaged this woman in conversation and encouraged her to sit with us. That didn't last long. After a few meals with us, the woman ironically declared, "You're crazy" and moved to another table. We laughed when that happened.

Laughter felt good and made the days less bleak. Laughter was also a way of relieving the tension caused by never knowing what would happen next or when we would finally be released.

After breakfast on my first full day in Brunswick, I wandered the hallway, waiting for maintenance personnel to finish washing the floor in the day room. When I was finally able to sit down in the room, a twenty-something "boy" named David sat down next to me. He introduced himself, asked my name and shook my hand.

"Can I ask you a question?" David asked. I smilingly nodded my assent.

"If you're wearing an orange shirt, does it mean I'll never see my mother again, or is that a delusion?"

Still smiling, I pointed out that it was certainly a delusion, and he shouldn't worry. How was I to know that at least once an hour of every single day, David would repeat some variation of the question? He'd constantly rush out of the day room to accost anyone walking by and ask:

"Will I be able to see my mother again?"

Often this question came in the form of a tantrum, like once when he started screaming and crying because an aide's shirt was decorated with a heart pattern.

"You're wearing hearts. Now I'll never be able to see my mother again."

Even some of the social workers eventually became short-tempered with him. David also ran to the phone in the day room every time it rang, once pushing me out of the way and almost knocking me over, in the hopes it would be his mother. Sometimes it was, and he'd exuberantly yell, *"Mommy!"* One day, when he hadn't heard from his mother in more than 24 hours, he grabbed the ringing phone and after a very excited *"MOMMY!"* let out a curdling scream: *"YOU BITCH!"* and started to berate her.

David's behavior was troubling to everyone in the ward—patients and staff alike. Given his age, it was surprising that he was in the geriatric ward at all. The ward that housed younger patients was at the end of our hallway on the other side of locked doors. David sometimes hung out by that door, talking through the glass to the boys and young men who were closer to his age.

Given everything I'd seen, it shouldn't have been a surprise that no one considered moving David until there was something of a crisis.

One day, David and his roommate got into an argument. David had told the roommate that he had a lover who was an Arab terrorist, and the roommate insisted David was a liar. The argument carried over into the day room where David became so angry that he threw a chair at his roommate. The flying chair passed too close to me for comfort.

While aides sought to calm David, I found the day nurse and inquired what I could do about feeling unsafe. The speed with which she called the chief of security indicated her eagerness to be rid of David. It seemed as if she'd just been waiting for an excuse to act. The security chief was quick to arrive, listened to my description of David's behavior and quickly had him transferred to the ward for youthful patients.

My guess is that David had been placed in the geriatric ward due to lack of beds. If I hadn't said something, who knows how long he'd have been kept there.

David wasn't the only "inmate" I felt threatened by. There was also Harriet—a middle-aged, wheelchair-bound woman missing most of her teeth. Whenever our paths crossed, she'd glare at me with the most malicious of expressions. She seemed to really dislike me, and I had no idea why. I wasn't certain how this sour woman felt about Evie when she said Evie looked familiar and asked if she had ever dealt crack. On another occasion, Harriet quickly wheeled herself into the dayroom to answer the ringing phone.

I heard her say, *"Linda's not here"* and hang up the phone.

When I pointed out that I was sitting right there, she angrily said, *"It was your son. You just saw him. You don't need to talk to him."*

I was stunned by her hostility. Harriet also had a habit of cackling—there is simply no other way to describe the sound of her laughter—as well as a tendency to berate other patients, making fun of their conditions and their appearance. Since she wasn't physically violent, these behaviors were allowed to continue regardless of how negatively they may have impacted the mental health of the other patients.

Another unusual "inmate" was a forty-something man named Bob who I met on my second morning. He sat next to me in the day room, and we were having such a nice conversation that I remember thinking, *"Maybe this won't be so bad."* Then the conversation turned to a discussion of the state of the world. At that point, Bob informed me that the government was using people's brain cells to run computers. Other theories he shared with me included Elvis Presley and Marilyn Monroe still being alive and hidden away. Bob's theories were not the most unsettling thing about him.

He was also too interested in touching or holding my hand—particularly disturbing since he had a skin condition on his hands. Staff members seemed to turn a blind eye to Bob's touching me, yet when I put my arm around Amy, I was told there was to be no physical contact between patients.

Bob was one of the people who went outside for supervised cigarette breaks twice a day. The outside areas where we could smoke were surrounded by fences (to keep us from escaping, of course). Bob was always being reprimanded for picking up trash or twigs and throwing them over the fences. His penchant for tossing things also led to a problem in the day room.

One morning, we entered the day room to find water stains on the wall next to the office. Bob had tossed water from a plastic cup. As a result, the water pitcher that was usually kept in the day room on a small table was removed. If we wanted a drink of water, we now had to get someone to unlock the dining room where there was another pitcher.

Bob was scolded as if he were a child who had done something wrong in class. I was acutely aware that the staff sometimes seemed to belittle patients. I also wondered if any of the professionals asked Bob why he felt the need to throw things. Doing so would be an example of reasonable mental health care, but nothing about Brunswick was reasonable.

Being around most of the inmates, with the exception of my small group of female friends, was not pleasant. One of the ways to "escape" was to take a shower. On one particular occasion, there wasn't any shampoo in my bin. When I asked for some, I was told to wash my hair with the soap in the dispenser on the shower wall. My long frizzy hair was going to be impossible to comb after that, but I had no choice.

Showered and frizzed, I headed back to my room where I discovered that a new patient had been admitted that morning and been assigned to my room. As I was putting the supplies I had taken to the shower back in my bin, this roommate noticed the green body wash. Mistaking it for alcohol-filled mouthwash, she grabbed it and tried to drink it.

This roommate and I shared the room for two nights. To say that her behavior was unsettling is probably an understatement. For most of the two days, she was asleep on the bed. She never came out of the room, not even for meals, which meant she wasn't eating. The rest of the time, she sat in a wheelchair in our room, staring into space or reading psalms from a small paper pamphlet.

The very first words she spoke to me were, "Wicked women go to hell." She didn't speak again until the next day when she asked if I was afraid of dying. Neither is a particularly comfortable conversation-starter. Then, she asked to borrow my hairbrush, and I recommended that she get a kit from the nurses' station. When she repeated the request, I gave the brush to her. Considering that she hadn't showered in the hospital, I never asked for her to return it.

Hanging around in my room while this woman was in residence was particularly uncomfortable, so I headed back to the day room. What else was there to do? I didn't have any books to read because the ones my son had brought me were deemed physically dangerous and taken away. Erik hadn't yet had an opportunity to bring me something acceptable.

The day room wasn't a very warm and welcoming place and could be downright unpleasant when patients were inevitably exhibiting their particular strange behaviors. One of the patients who exhibited such behaviors was the very obese man I had noticed at my first dinner. He often sat in the day room, reading a Bible and "talking" to Jesus. On a few occasions, he said, *"They crucified us both."*

While his ramblings were not particularly offensive, his odor was. He had been protesting something by refusing to shower and smelled horrible. In addition, he wore only two hospital gowns—one in the front and one in the back. If he was sitting with his knees apart, I was always afraid I'd see something I didn't want to see. One time he urinated in the chair he was sitting in. After that, I'd always ask one of the aides to wipe down his chair with disinfectant when he left the day room.

Having to cope with people whose behavior was so aberrant did not feel therapeutic to me. I am a nervous person by nature, and feeling uncomfortable and unsafe just made me more nervous. The professional staff did nothing to alleviate the feeling because they were either hard to find or seemed lost in their own heads.

Was the environment so toxic that even the staff had to adopt an escapist mentality to remain sane? Or were these simply underpaid, overworked government employees just putting in their hours until they could retire or find something better? Providing patients a safe, stable, and supportive environment should be a priority especially in mental hospitals. The staff and administration of Brunswick Hospital had apparently not received the memo or simply couldn't do anything about it.

The psychiatrist assigned to me was one of these seemingly lost professionals. I met her for about a half hour the day after I arrived, one of only three meetings during what would become almost a month of "incarceration." None of the meetings lasted any longer than that. At that first meeting, it became clear that this psychiatrist was, unfortunately, the victim of confirmation bias - the tendency to interpret information in a way that confirms one's beliefs while giving less consideration to alternative possibilities or to objectively examining facts.[35]

The psychiatrist knew that I was 65 years old, so the textbooks would consider me "geriatric." My history revealed that I was divorced, had lost a child and attempted suicide, and that my surviving child lived in Atlanta — more than 900 miles from my home. The psychiatrist was also, of course, aware of the textbook statistics revealing that suicide risk increases with age due to a lack of social interaction as well as the deaths of friends and loved ones over time.

Given these five simple facts about my history, her instantaneous judgement was that I was suffering from textbook geriatric depression. Later I learned she had said this almost verbatim to my son when he finally was afforded the opportunity to talk to her.

She never asked me any questions about my life that might have revealed alternative possibilities. In reality there wasn't much of a dialogue at all but rather a monologue with her telling me what was wrong with me without any real investigation. She never learned that I was not suffering from irritability, apathy, withdrawal, or changes in appetite which are among the most common symptoms of geriatric depression.

Although a suicide attempt can be an indication of depression, despair, or despondency, my attempt had not been prompted by any of these, but instead by the hope that I would be with Alan again when I died. In hindsight, that clearly wasn't a "sane" choice or plan, but it wasn't "textbook geriatric depression."

In addition, I had not been experiencing loneliness or alienation before Alan's death. I had been in a close and loving relationship with a man for a number of years. I was still teaching part-time and was the organizer of almost daily activities for a woman's group. The psychiatrist's confirmation bias can probably be best explained by *Psychology Today*: "Once we have formed a view, we embrace information that confirms that view while ignoring, or rejecting, information that casts doubt on it. Confirmation bias suggests that we don't perceive circumstances objectively."[35]

Any sort of investigation into my history would have revealed that even if I sometimes missed Erik, I was proud that he was living a full, productive, and happy life. It meant I had done my job as a parent. In fact, when Erik was handed to me in the hospital as a newborn, I'd looked at him and said, *"You're leaving me already."* I have always believed that a parent's job is to prepare a child to live independently and successfully on their own.

Kahil Gibran, a Lebanese-American artist, poet, and writer, said it best: "You are the bows from which your children as living arrows are sent forth." It is a parent's job to be a strong and stable bow and to offer all the nurturing necessary for the arrow to fly straight and true. I had succeeded with Erik. Because of that success, I was able to decide that he would be okay without me if I committed suicide. Even if he had lived close by, his independence and well-being would have brought me to the same conclusion. Do the psychology texts classify a parent who is content with the success of a child as someone with geriatric depression?

Even if the textbooks had accurately described all of my feelings, behaviors, personal analyses, and other traits as geriatric depression, simply slapping me with a label after a brief office visit does not seem at all conducive to providing effective therapy.

In any event, over the next several weeks, I wouldn't receive any actual therapy. The mental health system was only interested in shoving me into the medicine-driven gears on one side of the machine to be ground up until I could be spit out and discharged on the other side.

One question that the psychiatrist did bother to ask was whether I had slept the night before.

"No. I couldn't sleep because the woman in the room next to mine was screaming all night," was my response.

The psychiatrist said she'd write an order for sleeping pills for me.

In something right out of *Catch-22* by Joseph Heller, I was told the hospital couldn't legally force the woman who kept everyone on the floor awake all night to take sleeping pills or to be sedated. Instead, every patient who complained that the screams kept them awake was prescribed sleeping pills. Anyone who's experienced any extended period of sleeplessness can attest to a lack of sleep's effects on mental state.

So ,here we were, held hostage from sleep by a woman who herself was likely being held hostage in this facility. I am lucky I escaped with my sanity.

At this initial meeting with the psychiatrist, she prescribed several antidepressants and a sedative to help me sleep. I told her that, given the circumstances of my son's death, I didn't want to take that many pills. She sighed and agreed to begin with a trial of one antidepressant, Effexor, and the sedative.

Eventually, I asked that the sedative be discontinued. When I later asked the psychiatrist if the antidepressant or the blood pressure medications I had been newly prescribed at Brunswick were causing me to be sleepy, she blamed the weather.

The psychiatrist's total lack of knowledge about my background contributed to her having no respect for my opinions. When I was a child, dinner table conversations often included medications and their effects since my dad was a pharmacist and my uncle was an old-fashioned GP (general practitioner).

Later, I'd spent years dealing with the medications prescribed for Alan's psychological and physical problems and with the side effects those medications caused. I'd also been married to a biologist who'd spent his career investigating drugs, and I had even written a few books about alternative medicine, so I had learned a thing or two about pills. The psychiatrist had learned none of that about me and probably wouldn't have cared about it even if she had known.

In scenes reminiscent of *One Flew Over the Cuckoo's Nest*, twice a day we were told to line up to get our medication. Echoes of Belgian singer/songwriter Jacques Brel deeply and angrily intoning, "Next, next./ I stand on endless naked lines/Of the following and the followed. Next. Next," rang in my head.

Patient after patient walked up to the medication dispensing window, open just wide enough to accommodate the passage of a medicine cup. Unlike Brel, we were neither naked nor angry, although on one occasion a man did arrive wearing nothing but his underpants. Patients lined up along the hallway walls—no chairs allowed—and proceeded docilely, some even eagerly, awaiting the "magic elixir" that would obliterate physical and/or psychic pain — or perhaps just help them deal with the hospital.

At night, dispensing of medicine was a little different. Night medication for almost all patients included sleeping pills, which meant a guaranteed temporary reprieve from the misery of incarceration. Patients would, therefore, rush to be at the front of the line—even the women in wheelchairs. The "three witches" and I laughed as we watched what we called the "wheelchair races."

Day or night, when each patient arrived at the window, the dispensing nurse would consult a notebook that included a photo of the patient with a list of the prescribed medications. I had arrived at Brunswick during off hours on a weekend, and my picture had not been taken. In fact, my picture was not taken until three days before my discharge. Because of this, the nurse simply asked my date of birth in order to confirm my identity. Only if I had been refused medication because of the lack of a picture would the situation have been more fit for inclusion in *Catch-22*.

Almost every person on the line counted the pills and confirmed the pills' purposes with the nurse. Because many of them had been in psychiatric wards before, they had come to mistrust the process of dispensing medication. Frequently, the dispensing nurses called out the names of the drugs as they gave them to patients. So much for patient privacy and adherence to HIPAA!

Another seeming violation of HIPAA occurred one morning. My psychiatrist was the same woman who was working with Amy. After breakfast, Amy became very upset about the quality of the food at the hospital and complained loudly and at length. The psychiatrist happened to be standing next to me at the door to the dining room and said, *"She is really not a well woman."* Even if it were true, in addition to being very disrespectful to Amy, it was totally unprofessional and, to a lawyer, probably a HIPAA violation.

No matter which pills were included in our little plastic cups, every single patient received Colace twice a day to alleviate the constipation often caused by psychotropic drugs and always caused by opioid pain-killers. Many of the patients suffered from chronic pain, a condition which no doubt contributed to their depression and anxiety. Unfortunately, the Colace didn't help me much as the bathroom situation was far from hospitable.

Each bathroom was a small, dimly lit square with a sink, a toilet, and a shower stall with a plastic curtain. For whatever reason, there was no mirror. Despite there being a designated bathroom for each sex, everyone used both in order to get into a bathroom when it was needed. In addition, the men's room was much cleaner because one of the male patients who was obsessive compulsive cleaned it several times a day.

There was no sign on the men's room door, but a sign on the ladies' room door proclaimed in large letters, "KNOCK FIRST AND WAIT BEFORE OPENING." Nonetheless, people, including one man, walked in on me three times.

Far more awkward, and even a little eerie, was an encounter I had one day after I had urinated. After washing my hands, I turned and opened the door to walk out of the bathroom. At that moment, a female patient came out from behind the shower curtain with the tiniest smile on her face. She had been in the bathroom with me the entire time I was using the toilet, but I was completely unaware. Totally stunned, I didn't utter a word, but I did inform the day nurse. The nurse's reaction? A bemused shake of her head.

Given all of this, it's no surprise that the Colace didn't help me much: it's too hard to unclench your bowels when you worry that at any moment someone will walk in on you. I wasn't the only one having trouble moving my bowels. Several of us requested milk of magnesia in addition to the Colace in the hopes that would help. While Colace was prescribed as a matter of protocol, milk of magnesia wasn't available without a doctor's orders, so we just had to wait.

Klonopin was another drug that almost all of the patients were given. This was one of the drugs that Alan had become dependent on and that had contributed to his overdose. Everything I've read indicates that Klonopin, a benzodiazepine which is used to treat anxiety and schizophrenia, "may be habit forming." For this reason, the literature points out that those who have exhibited addiction to drugs or alcohol should not be prescribed Klonopin. It is also not recommended for those with a history of depression or suicidal thoughts or behavior and is considered particularly dangerous in older adults because the sedative effects last longer in older people.[36]

Addiction, depression, and suicide attempts were the very conditions that had led to the hospitalization of many of the patients in the geriatric ward! Yet, for some reason, Klonopin was commonly prescribed.

On the second evening of my confinement, I was given four pills instead of just the Effexor (for depression) and Colace I expected, so I asked what the other two pills were. The dispensing nurse said one was for my GERD (gastroesophageal reflux disease) and the other was to help me sleep. I had been taking medication for reflux for years and knew quite well that I had only been prescribed one pill a day. *"I took my GERD pill this morning,"* I replied.

The nurse insisted that I needed it that night, too. Rather than risk being considered uncooperative, I took the pills.

The next morning, I felt so drugged that I could barely open my eyes. I subsequently refused any pills except the Effexor and Colace.

Eventually, another nurse in the dispensary told me that the extra pills I had been given were Xyprexa (an antipsychotic sometimes used in conjunction with antidepressants) and Remeron (an antidepressant that is used as a sleeping medication because of its sedative effects).

They had been prescribed by the psychiatrist without any discussion with me or any explanation. In reality, this violates the regulations of the New York State Office of Mental Health which state, "Medications may be used only for therapeutic purposes, and the purpose and possible side effects, along with alternative treatments available, must be explained to you."[37] No one had even discussed the side effects of the one antidepressant drug I'd agreed to take when I initially met with the psychiatrist.

When I was finally able to talk to the psychiatrist again, she told me the pills that she had prescribed (without consulting me) would help me sleep. I explained that those pills made me feel like a zombie, which was why I refused to take them. I also again pointed out that my lack of sleep the first night had been caused by the screams of the woman in the room next to mine, and not by any inner turmoil on my part.

I also refused to take increasingly high doses of antidepressants because throughout the decades when Alan was treated with psychotropic drugs, I'd learned how many negative side effects these drugs have. Instead of trying to assuage my fears, understand my concerns, or change my medication, the psychiatrist simply labeled me as "resistant to therapy."

When taking medication is equated to therapy, it should be painfully obvious that the system is horrifically broken.

Labeling me as "resistant" was one of the reasons that my stay in the hospital was longer than that of other patients diagnosed with major depression. No one seemed to notice or care that avoiding drugs was partially a response to my son's fatal overdose, and certainly no one paused to wonder what the physiological repercussions of the "pill therapy" might be.

Although "therapeutic" drugs were readily and liberally administered for psychiatric uses, medication for physical maladies was very hard to obtain. The blood pressure pills I'd been taking for years were not available in the hospital's pharmacy, and the hospital couldn't (or wouldn't) get them. The replacement medication I was given wasn't doing a great job of controlling my pressure, which the daily vitals checks showed was going up and down erratically.

The medical doctor decided to double the blood pressure medication dosage. One afternoon I was so sleepy that I couldn't keep my eyes open and had to take a nap. I wondered if the increased dose of blood pressure medication had caused this. When I requested the literature about the pill's side effects, the dispensing nurse said, *"You can get that from the pharmacy. Next."*

What pharmacy? Brunswick's pharmacy? The corner pharmacy? *"How,"* I wondered, *"am I supposed to accomplish that when I'm locked in here?"*

Fortunately, the dispensing nurse on the next shift, who was one of the few true professionals I encountered at Brunswick, got the literature for me. Indeed, one of the listed side effects of this new blood pressure medication was drowsiness.

The next morning, I knocked repeatedly on the locked office door in the day room until the medical doctor looked up from his paperwork. At first, I had to speak to him through the glass panel on the locked door. Finally, one of the PAs opened the door, and I explained my situation to the doctor. His reply—without looking up from his paperwork—was that he hadn't increased my dose. Since the nurse who had dispensed the pills was standing right behind me, I turned to her and she confirmed that the dose had been doubled.

The morning after that, I received the original dose, which we already knew would be ineffective at controlling my blood pressure, and was told that my son could bring my prescription medications from home. When my son Erik had originally brought my prescription with him the day I was admitted, he was told I could not have those pills in the hospital. Now that someone had decided I could have them, Erik was out of the country on a business trip, and I couldn't get my medication until he returned more than a week later and only a few days before my discharge. What would have happened if my reaction to the new blood pressure medication had been more severe?

Decisions about patient medication seemed to revolve primarily around keeping patients "safe," which mostly translated to "docile enough not to do themselves or others any harm." In spite of the psychiatrist's insistence that people could not be forced to take medication, on two occasions I witnessed patients being forcibly sedated.

Apparently, forced sedation is acceptable once a patient becomes violent enough that they are a danger to themselves or others.

In one case, a young woman had caused a huge commotion because she refused to let the aids remove the underwires (potential weapons) from her bra. Sadly, this woman spoke only Creole, so her feelings of isolation, frustration and possibly even fear were exacerbated by the language barrier. She started kicking and screaming, and everyone in the day room rushed into the hall to watch the activity in the women's room. Eventually the woman was put in restraints and sedated. "Show" over; boredom resumed.

David was the other patient who was forcibly sedated. One day he was more than usually upset about his mother and was waiting for her to call. As time passed and she still hadn't called, he began ranting and threw a book across the day room. When the PAs tried to calm him, he began shoving them, and the decision was made to sedate him.

Sedation, anti-anxiety medication, and antidepressants were all dispensed freely at Brunswick. Psycho*pharmacology* was clearly the hospital's priority with psycho*therapy* a distant second.

I was in the hospital for two weeks before I met with the psychologist who had been assigned to me, yet I saw the psychiatrist and was prescribed medication almost immediately upon my arrival. When I finally did meet with this psychologist, most of the session was devoted to her learning my background. There was no opportunity for the kind of conversation that aims to remedy a patient's psychic disturbance.

In the 21 days I was hospitalized, I saw the psychologist for a total of about 1 hour, the psychiatrist for a total of about 90 minutes, and the medical doctor for about 20 minutes.

Each patient was also assigned a social worker whose primary responsibility was coordinating "care," especially as it related to discharge. My social worker managed to make me feel as if I were a child who didn't have the brains or ability to run my own life. I certainly never felt that she treated me with either respect or dignity. The last component in my "therapy" consisted of various group sessions.

"Art therapy" was scheduled once a week in the day room. When each of these sessions started, we were handed a clip board and asked to sign a piece of paper which indicated that we had attended. Even people sitting in the chairs around the perimeter of the day room and not participating were asked to sign. We were told that, by signing, we would be "given credit" for attending.

During the sessions, there was never any discussion of what we were doing, why we were doing it, or of what our art work might reveal about us. Being involved in an art project was nice, but mostly because it was slightly better than doing nothing at all. Probably it simply checked some bureaucratic box that ensured we weren't being treated cruelly or unusually and that we were receiving sanctioned "treatment" for our illnesses.

The "therapy" usually involved coloring, which did have a calming effect as we concentrated on outlining and staying in the lines. During one art session, there were various sized square and rectangular pieces of colored paper on the table. We were told to paste the small papers onto a larger piece of paper in order to create a picture. I made a tree, which I referred to as my "cubist period."

"Music therapy" was also offered once every ten days or so. During these sessions we listened to CDs as a group. The group facilitator offered a choice of rock or jazz, but there was no discussion. At least there was some consistency in the complete lack of real therapy.

Along with activity-based therapy sessions, a weekly group therapy session was held. Even this was less than helpful. During group therapy, we often filled out questionnaires, but, consistent with the theme of simply going through the motions, there was rarely any discussion of our responses. Discussion that would have been helpful to any one patient was difficult because the group included addicts, diagnosed psychotics, schizophrenics, and depressed people. Although the problems and needs within the group were vastly different, the questions and lists we were given focused on how to avoid the pitfalls that could lead to relapse into addiction.

One-on-one therapy would have been far more effective as it could have been tailored to individual needs. When I discussed this with the social worker in charge of recreational therapy, she told me she understood my discontent, but pointed out that there was no budget for more individualized programs. Furthermore, the limited budget didn't allow for patients with different conditions and different needs to be separated into different facilities or wards. My son Alan had struggled his whole life with the system's inability to address his differences, and now I seemed to be suffering the same fate.

To add insult to the depraved situation that I found myself in, questions about hospital conditions or treatment were usually met with some variation of *"If you question or resist, your stay in the hospital will be longer."* Those words would come back to haunt me as my efforts to maintain my sanity or look out for my physical health were viewed as "resistance to treatment."

My release was postponed — twice. I think there may be a method to this madness. Because patients are so frustrated by delayed release, when they are finally "sprung," all they feel is relief. They have no energy left to pursue any redress of their grievances.

My inability to get any staff member to respond to my personal, individual needs reminded me of the way prisoners are tortured until they acquiesce to some falsehood. In this case, the falsehood was that the environment was therapeutic, everything was fine, and I was getting better. The torture was simply the act of keeping me in the hospital.

So there we all were: screaming patients who kept people awake at night, delusional patients who pestered others with repeated ramblings, cruel patients who verbally abused others. And all of us participated in ineffective group therapy that, at best, catered to the lowest common denominator or, more realistically, was just ticking boxes.

Ultimately, the only real "therapy" that could efficiently be provided to such a diverse group was medication or, more accurately, suppression. Several different staff members actually told us on separate occasions that the hospital's only job was to medicate us. And medicate us they did.

Over-reliance on medication and a lack of adequate or relevant counseling weren't the only deficits in treatment. Despite the commonly held belief that a healthy mind requires a healthy body, there was absolutely no exercise program. When we asked about exercise, we were told that there was an exercise DVD for our use, but the DVD player wasn't working. A game room on the lower level of the hospital had ping pong and air hockey tables, but we were only given access to that room once in the time I was a patient. On that occasion, Amy was even able to persuade the very disheveled lady to join us and played ping pong with her.

Sometimes, patients were allowed to go outside for 15 minutes, which would be their only opportunity to get exposure to direct sunlight. That happened only four times in my 21 days there. Fortunately for me, being a smoker meant that I got more outside time than others when I went on the twice-daily smoke breaks we were offered. Twisted, isn't it, that one has to engage in unhealthy behavior in order to be rewarded with sunlight and fresh air?

Eventually, it became clear that the hospital was falsifying records indicating that physical activity was being provided. When we were told to sign in for activities even if we weren't participating, we complied so we could be considered cooperative. Thinking that a depressed person wouldn't participate, I always made sure to sign in and take part in the activity.

Toward the end of my hospitalization, I realized that I was signing in for an exercise program when the activity being conducted was something else entirely. A number of the sheets I signed had probably also indicated some kind of physical activity was being conducted.

In the same healthy body/healthy mind category, nutrition at Brunswick Hospital could be politely described as "not great." Our meals were heavy on starches (both potatoes and corn at one meal, for instance). Few non-starchy vegetables were provided, and those that were appeared to be canned, not fresh. "Salad" consisted only of iceberg lettuce. Sandwiches, the standard lunch offering, were filled with processed meats. Breakfast was scrambled eggs that were obviously made from dehydrated eggs. Other breakfast choices consisted of oatmeal or sometimes pancakes.

Every morning, pre-packed plastic bowls of generic fruit loops and cocoa puffs were offered and eagerly consumed by patients — unless their trays indicated they were diabetic. Fresh fruit was always served, but some days it was a banana at all three meals.

I had been put on a no-sugar diet because my blood sugar tested a little high when I was admitted, but I was still being served lots of heavily processed carbohydrates which any nutritionist with even basic training would know has a direct correlation to increased blood sugar.

The yogurt I had for breakfast every day was sweetened with aspartame, even though its safety has been in question for some time: studies link it to vision problems and headaches.[38]

When I pointed out that aspartame worsens my flatulence, the nutritionist agreed but said that the artificially sweetened yogurt was the only type available. With so many yogurt products on the market, I have to wonder why this was so. Perhaps the yogurt available in the hospital was obtained at less cost? But shouldn't the patient's well-being have been the primary concern?

Even though I was leery of being considered a difficult patient, I refused the yogurt and was offered the cold cereal, which was nothing but processed grain (carbohydrate) and tons of added sugar. When I refused the cold cereal, the nutritionist decided to give me half of a turkey sandwich on whole wheat bread for breakfast.

It seemed that my only choices were either worsening my blood sugar with processed foods or worsening my flatulence with artificial sweeteners. One morning, I ate the turkey sandwich out of desperation and hunger. Another morning, I buttered the bread and ate that, leaving the turkey behind.

Eventually, I asked for the artificially sweetened yogurt. Many of my problems with the food could have been solved if Erik had been allowed to bring in food. Absolutely no outside foods—not even snacks—could be brought into the hospital.

Excessive restrictions, poor nutrition, lack of exercise, and boredom combined to make my life at Brunswick miserable. A great deal of my misery came from loss of self-worth and self-esteem. Nothing about me as a person was valued or even recognized. In addition, the institutional environment that was supposed to be therapeutic was actually anxiety-producing.

I didn't feel physically safe.

I couldn't predict what might happen.

I couldn't understand things that did happen.

Perhaps what bothered me most was the feeling that control over my life had been completely stripped away, leaving me feeling helpless. Ironically, depression studies indicate that a person's reduced feeling of control and lack of options in a situation "can further add to the depression."[39]

Realizing how miserable I was and seeing a deterioration in my mental condition during my time at Brunswick, Erik discussed various possibilities with hospital staff. This led to my being given a marble-covered composition notebooks so that I could keep a journal of my experiences.

Unfortunately, patients weren't allowed pens. The one pencil I was given had to be frequently sharpened, which meant finding an aide who could take the pencil into the office to sharpen it and then bring it back.

What should have been an additional therapeutic avenue turned into yet another form of tilting at windmills and a source of anxiety and frustration. It gave me a sense of how Alan must have felt about the slant board. Not surprisingly, writing in the journal never became part of my routine.

All of these things may have contributed to an incident that I believe extended my hospital stay.

One morning, approximately ten days into my hospitalization, Harriet the toothless, wheelchair-bound woman was cackling even more loudly than usual at breakfast and taunting one of the women at her table. The other patients at the table tried to get Harriet to stop, but she kept cackling and making fun of people. When breakfast ended, we had our cigarette break and then headed to the day room for art "therapy."

The social worker in charge of the session was playing music on a CD player. At this session, while Harriet cackled and loud music played,

Bob started to rant that he didn't belong in the hospital and had been sent there simply for throwing a ball against the wall of his group home. He went on and on, repeating the story to everyone within earshot.

I have never liked noise. I've never been able to study or write with music playing. And here I was surrounded by noise as I attempted to put together pieces of colored paper that would become a flower pot with a large tulip in it. Harriet was cackling, Bob was ranting *and* music was playing. It was all too much for me, and I ran back to my room, crying.

The aide who was stationed at the end of the hall near my room came in to comfort me. She asked me if I wanted to pray to which I responded, *"There's no one to pray to."* She went on to say that the Lord is always there for us and then told me to rest. Although touched by her kindness, her "preaching" struck me as inappropriate for mental health personnel. I'm certain the other mental health professionals at Brunswick were informed of my behavior and construed it as "impulsive," which was one of the reasons that I was not allowed to return home sooner.

Later that day, I went back to the day room and glued the paper flower into a paper pot. By this time, Bob's medication had been changed, and he became quieter. Harriet continued to glare at me from her wheelchair, but a new patient had been admitted, which gave Harriet someone else to focus on.

The new arrival, Molly, was a very thin fifty-something woman who spoke with an affected upper class voice. She paced the day room all day long, talking to herself. The only time her monologue ceased was when she returned to her room to change her clothing—which she did several times a day. Every time Molly came into the day room in a new outfit, Harriet would snarl something like, *"What's the matter with you? Why do you have to keep changing clothes?"* or she'd cackle *"Here comes the prima donna."*

The days passed until Erik came back from his business trip to Germany, and I had his visits to look forward to. One evening, the social worker sat with us and said that my release would be in two days. What relief and happiness I felt!

Subsequently, the psychiatrist and the hospital's discharge group considered my case and decided to postpone my release because I had been "resistant to treatment, impulsive, and argumentative." I had made it a point to participate in everything so that no one could claim I was depressed, uncooperative, or non-compliant.

Apparently, asking that my drug regimen be revised meant that I was "resistant to treatment." YES, I was — and continue to be — resistant to taking drugs. Given Alan's history, that shouldn't have been surprising.

Of course, since I later learned that the hospital records incorrectly indicated that Alan had died in a motor vehicle accident, the reasoning behind my resistance wouldn't have crossed their minds. How such misinformation about my son's death got into my records, I'll never know.

I suspect that I was considered impulsive partly because of my being reduced to tears by all the noise during art therapy. The label of "impulsive" is, however, surprising since I'd been told that it was precisely the detailed planning of my suicide attempt that meant that I was "high risk." As for the claim that I was "argumentative," I was floored.

"Ask any of the aides; they all like me," I said.

The response was, *"They like everyone."*

In retrospect, I should have said, *"The aides will tell you I never argued with anyone,"* but I don't think fast on my feet, especially when I am upset. In addition, I am not by nature an assertive person; "Peace at any price" might be my motto. In fact, Erik often calls me a "wuss" because I do not stand up for myself. Although I am opinionated about certain things and may hotly debate social or political issues, none of that came up in the hospital.

When I was discharged, I hugged the one professional — a nurse — whose competence and common sense could never be questioned. When she said "goodbye," she also whispered in my ear, *"Watch what you say; you don't belong here."* I imagine any of the aides — all of whom treated patients with respect and genuine concern and most of whom I was quite friendly with — would have made similar comments.

Time and again, my questioning of or objection to the methodologies employed at the institution were viewed as resistance and argumentativeness. Yet New York State regulations include the statement, "You have a right to object to any form of care and treatment, and to appeal decisions with which you disagree."[40]

It was only after I was released from Brunswick that I discovered the "basic treatment plan shall include a statement of the goals of treatment, appropriate programs, treatment or therapies to be undertaken to meet the goals and a specific timetable for reviewing progress."[41]

No one ever told me or discussed with me the goals of my treatment.

It's my impression that the only goal was to "stabilize" my mood with medication so that I would be unlikely to make another attempt on my life.

In addition, I did not "… have the opportunity to participate as fully as [I was] able in establishing and revising [my] individual treatment plan" as stated in the NYS Office of Mental Health's requirements for Psychiatric Centers.[42] The law also states that patients have the right "to ask that the plan be revised."

It is ironic that those who are apprehended for criminal offenses are read their rights before being arrested, but mental patients, at least at Brunswick, are apparently not informed of their rights.

Mental hospitals are aware that their patients are not likely to know the laws, so they can afford to be lax about them. If patients do try to to exercise what they perceive as their rights, they experience negative consequences.

When family members know or take the time to learn the rules, they are rarely inclined to pursue legal channels. Erik and the son of another patient did discuss the possibility of a lawsuit, but neither did anything about it. Patients and family members usually just want to put the whole experience behind them.

Even bad times can end and, finally, I was told that I was going to be released. I was also told that after discharge, I was required to attend an outpatient program called a "partial program" sponsored by Mercy Hospital. This program met from 10 A.M. to 4 P.M. five days a week for six weeks. This requirement didn't make me happy as it would continue to curtail my life and take control away from me. Furthermore, I doubted it would prove any more beneficial than "lock up" had been.

Erik convinced me that it was important and "iced the cake" by pointing out that the program included a "therapy dog." He knew how much I loved animals.

The morning of my release arrived, and Erik and I headed to the diner near my apartment for corned beef hash — nothing has ever tasted so good!

The next morning, we went to an intake meeting for the partial program. A lovely young social worker read my charts and looked at me strangely when I explained that I was reluctant to take psychotropic medication because of Alan's overdose.

She looked at me quizzically and consulted the chart again. Then she told me that the information she had on the papers indicated Alan's cause of death was MVA — motor vehicle accident.

How can I be expected to trust what any health professionals tell me when they make egregious mistakes like that? How do I even know that my involuntary commitment to Brunswick was not affected by the false information? Would Winthrop's mental health evaluators have viewed Alan's death from a motor vehicle accident as less of a "sane" motivation for my suicide attempt than his death by a prescription drug overdose?

At 10 A.M. on the second day after I left Brunswick, I reported to the facility that housed the outpatient program. It was almost as drab as Brunswick, but the lunches were a lot better: a sandwich, drink, and fresh fruit. When I met the people in my group, I realized that, just like in Brunswick, they had a wide assortment of issues. One extremely talkative woman suffered from bipolar disorder. One very young man was struggling with depression and another man was schizophrenic. A couple of the men abused drugs and/or alcohol.

It appeared that a couple of the participants were required to attend the partial program by New York State's Assertive Community Treatment (ACT) law. This legislation ensures that people diagnosed with severe mental illness who have had multiple hospitalizations receive rehabilitation, case management, and support services. The aim is to give people the tools necessary to live outside of hospitals: to obtain and maintain housing, employment, relationships, and relief from symptoms and medication's side effects.

Ultimately, the intent is that people receiving the services are integrated into their natural community. Much of what was discussed in the partial program on a daily basis involved the basic life skills these people needed and was not relevant to me. In addition, a lot of emphasis was placed on helping recovering addicts stay clean and sober.

As irrelevant as these two focus areas were to me, the program ultimately proved to be helpful.

After Erik returned to Atlanta, knowing that I had to go to the partial program gave me a reason to get up, get dressed, and get out of my apartment each day.

In this program, the art therapy included discussion of the drawings and collages we made. We also wrote journals which we shared with the group and which the group leader commented on. A few afternoons included doing exercises as demonstrated on a DVD.

The therapy dog turned out to belong to the art therapist's wheelchair-bound daughter and only came in one day to show us how he could be asked to bring various items—including a tissue—to the girl.

The most useful part of the program, though, was instruction in stress management which centered on mindfulness techniques. We learned that stress and anxiety arise when we experience regrets about the past or worry about the future. Keeping our minds centered on the present moment helps to hold stress and anxiety at bay.

The techniques we were taught included controlled breathing exercises and counting objects we could see, hear, feel and smell. These techniques continue to be useful to me on an almost daily basis.

Far less useful were the afternoon sessions when we went around the room, each of us reading a section of a handout that was usually devoted to information about substance abuse. It was very difficult for me to sit still and listen to several group members' labored reading, and the content was totally irrelevant to my life.

After three weeks, the social workers assigned to my group decided it was time for me to graduate. Perhaps they thought that I wouldn't gain any further benefit from the sessions and that there were people far more in need of the program. I was still required to see the program's psychologist on a bi-weekly basis and to see its psychiatrist monthly.

Sessions with the psychologist were not very helpful. He was a very warm and caring man who I enjoyed talking with, but he acknowledged that there wasn't much he could do to help me. Grieving is, after all, a process.

The real goal of having a psychologist was to give me someone to call if I became suicidal, which I haven't to this day and probably never will again. No matter how painful my grief, I always remember that there are people in my life who I love deeply, good friends who are always willing to talk, and a job that I love. That's more than a lot of people ever have.

The psychiatrist I was assigned in the partial program continued to prescribe antidepressant medications which I reluctantly continued to take. After two months, this psychiatrist was transferred to another post, and I was assigned to someone else. At the first session with the new psychiatrist, my history was reviewed and then he launched into a rather long monologue about his difficulties with his own children.

Although this was awkward and not ideal given my history with Alan, I dutifully returned a month later. This time, there was a nameplate on the desk, and I discovered that the man was not a psychiatrist but a psychiatric nurse practitioner.

These practitioners hold either a master's or doctoral degree rather than the M.D. degree that psychiatrists have. They receive extensive training in physical and mental health assessment, the diagnosis of mental health conditions, psychopharmacology and psychotherapy. The man was obviously quite qualified, but I was surprised no one had thought to mention his credentials when I was reassigned. It struck me as disingenuous and not in keeping with a patient's right to be fully informed about treatment.

Still, I returned for a third session. I walked in and sat down.

The psychiatric nurse asked, *"Are you feeling ok?"*

I said, *"Yes."*

He renewed my prescription and sent me on my way. A five-minute session and another prescription. That was the last I saw of him. What was the point of returning? Should I continue to get pills that I really didn't want to be taking and honestly didn't believe were helping me?

I did continue taking the antidepressant for a few more months under the supervision of my internist but eventually decided that taking them was pointless.

I had a right to grieve.

Some days that meant I could barely get out of bed, didn't get dressed, and didn't go out. I had a right to feel my pain and to express it in whatever way it manifested: to weep and scream, to kick doors, to rail against malevolent fate. Still, I continued to work and socialize. Keeping busy was, for me, the best medicine.

Sometimes I think that maybe I wasn't learning to cope or to deal with my grief. Perhaps I was just keeping so busy that I didn't have time or even energy to confront my pain.

I went back to teaching part-time and returned to organizing events for my women's social group. I joined a support group for bereaved parents, COPE (Connecting Our Paths Eternally), which provided a safe place to talk about my grief and my guilt without fear of being judged. Here I often cried my heart out.

I was also blessed by the continued friendship of Evie, one of the "three witches" I'd met at Brunswick Hospital. We'd been roommates on her last night in the hospital and, like teenagers at a slumber party, we gabbed all night. After her discharge, I found she had left a note for me on my shelf.

She told me how much she admired my devotion to Alan. According to her I was "the strongest woman she knew." She'd included her email address and phone number, and I contacted her as soon as I got home. Over the next two years, we became more than just good friends.

To Evie, who felt her family had abandoned her when she needed them most, I was almost a surrogate mother. In Evie's own words, *"I love you like a best friend, but I also have a love for you like a daughter would for a mother."* Evie felt that I was supporting and helping her in the way she wished her mother could have.

We would meet at an area park three times a week to walk and talk or we'd go out for dinner, sharing our pain and our fears. We could talk about the days we couldn't get out of bed, the need for naps, the constant eating of junk food with no fear of judgement. There was true and deep empathy between us. And somehow we always managed to laugh. Who else in the world would laugh with us about suicide attempts or depression?

Evie would ask so many questions about Alan. She was the only one who wasn't fearful of doing that. Even the other mothers in COPE didn't ask, fearful perhaps of being intrusive or of opening deep wounds. Evie's incredible warmth, generosity and humor helped me get through the hardest days of my life, but my love for her could not alleviate the physical and psychic pain she herself suffered.

Tragically, two years after her discharge from Brunswick, Evie became another statistic when she succeeded in taking her own life.

The back pain Evie experienced was not adequately controlled by the high doses of pain medication she was prescribed. Her fear that the tumor would return again and, this time, be inoperable was not alleviated by the anti-anxiety medications she was prescribed. Her depression over having had to give up her active lifestyle and lucrative career was not lifted by the antidepressants she was prescribed.

Hours and hours in therapy and days of incarceration at Brunswick had done nothing to make her feel that her life was worth living. Evie was briefly confined to a different psychiatric facility following a suicide threat. That facility discharged her after declaring that she was not at risk.

To add to her burden, in addition to her back pain, Evie was diagnosed as severely anemic and told she needed intravenous iron infusions. Living on the limited income provided by disability insurance, Evie was heavily in debt and couldn't afford more medical treatments.

Just three months after being diagnosed as "not at risk" and released from a 72-hour psychiatric hold, Evie committed suicide.

The system — mental, medical, economic — had failed completely.

SUICIDE RECIDIVISM

Anyone who listens to the radio, reads a newspaper, or has a Facebook account, knows of the suicides of Seymour Hoffman, Robin Williams, Kate Spade, Anthony Bourdain… the list goes on and on. How many people, however, know that in 2010, four years before his death by hanging, Robin Williams had slit his wrists in a failed suicide attempt?

Long ago, it was believed that someone who had a failed suicide attempt would not make a repeat attempt. History has shown this to be blatantly untrue.

In fact, there is an especially high risk of a repeat attempt in the first six months after an initial attempt. One study revealed that "The rate of suicide in the self-harm patient population is up to 100 times higher than that of the general population."[43] Another study in Great Britain reported that patients who have more than one suicide attempt have approximately double the risk of yet another suicide attempt compared to those who have made only one attempt.[44]

Although repeat suicide attempts have been studied for more than 30 years, no prevention plan has had a significant effect on the incidence of those attempts. A 2011 study reported, "People who attempt suicide are at high risk of further repetition. However, no interventions have been shown to be effective in reducing repetition in this group of patients."[45]

It's not just repeat suicide attempts that have stymied professionals. An article in the World Psychiatric Association's journal in 2014 concluded that "researchers and clinicians alike have been stumped in the quest to decrease suicide rates... [The] predictors simply do not work well, especially in identifying short-term risk."[46]

One "predictor" that clinicians have traditionally used to assess risk is the presence of "suicidal ideation." This approach is problematic because the term is ambiguously defined. Sometimes suicidal ideation is defined as the presence of both thoughts of suicide and suicidal behaviors. Sometimes, suicidal ideation refers to actual plans to commit suicide or voicing the wish to die.

Furthermore, statistical analysis does not support a correlation between suicide attempts and suicidal ideation. An analysis of hundreds of studies (meta-analysis) published in January 2019*[BJPsych]* showed that 60 percent of people who had committed suicide had not expressed suicidal ideation when specifically asked about it, and 80 percent of people who attempted suicide had not expressed suicidal ideation when questioned by a general practitioner.

This data supports the conclusion that "the presence or absence of suicide-related thoughts or expressions of suicidal ideation does not predict later suicide."[47] The same study also revealed that in-depth questioning about suicidal thoughts and plans is associated with an increased risk of incorrectly assessing people as at risk for suicide. The lead investigators in one study conclude, "...suicidal ideation is not sensitive enough to be very helpful as a stand-alone screening test ..."[48]

Another reason for the failure to curb repeat suicide attempts may be that, for many years, the prevention of suicide and the efforts to treat those who had attempted it revolved around diagnosing and treating depression. Once again, however, the statistics do not support the theory.

For instance, a 2014 article in *World Psychiatry* reports that only about 10 percent of people who commit suicide in the U.S. "have an identifiable mental disorder," and only about 5 to 10 percent of those with unipolar depression commit suicide. The rate had been believed to be higher when the statistics came primarily from in-patient sampling. "Thus, suicidal behavior does not appear to be an intrinsic dimension of any particular psychiatric disorder."[49]

Not only is a diagnosis of depression not helpful in preventing suicide, but treatment of depression usually relies on antidepressants, which may actually increase the risk of suicide. Some studies have shown that the Selective Serotonin Reuptake Inhibitors (SSRIs) commonly used to treat depression are associated with an increased suicide risk; one study reported that in children and adolescents the risk of suicidality and aggression doubled.[50]

The Food and Drug Administration believed the association between suicide and antidepressants in children and young adults was credible enough to merit a strong warning for these populations in 2004. One study contradicting the FDA's conclusion was based on data obtained from the National Institute of Mental Health's Treatment for Adolescents With Depression Study as well as from the drug companies Wyeth and Eli Lilly and Co.[51] Unfortunately, the pharmaceutical industry has a reputation for corrupting research into the risk and efficacy of antidepressants.

This history was detailed in a 2015 article in *Scientific American* entitled "Many Antidepressant Studies Found Tainted by Pharma Company Influence."[52] Significant evidence of suicide risk was presented in March 2019 in the journal *Psychotherapy and Psychosomatics*. The authors reported that when they re-analyzed the FDA safety summaries, they compared the number of suicides among patients receiving various antidepressants with those who received placebos. They "found evidence that the rate of (attempted) suicide was about 2.5 times higher" in antidepressant users than in those using a placebo.[53]

Pharmaceutical companies' interference in studies is just one of the reasons that the efficacy of antidepressants is hotly debated. According to an article published by the National Institutes of Health, "Antidepressants are supposed to work by fixing a chemical imbalance, specifically, a lack of serotonin in the brain. Ttheir supposed effectiveness is the primary evidence for the chemical imbalance theory. But analyses of *both* the published data and the unpublished data that were hidden by drug companies reveals that most (if not all) of the benefits are due to the placebo effect."[54]

The inconclusive connection between depression and suicide and the potential negative effects of antidepressant medications on those with psychiatric disorders may well be the reasons that many mental health professionals and researchers now advocate that suicidal behavior should be studied "independently of any associated psychiatric disorder."[55]

For many psychiatrists dealing with depressed patients or patients with suicidal ideation, drugs are still the go-to choice. Sadly, at Brunswick Hospital and, I suspect, at many psychiatric facilities, drugs are also still the treatment of choice.

Patients are involuntarily committed as Evie and I were when they are considered to be a danger to themselves or to society.[56] During such commitment, alleviating this presumed immediate danger usually involves the use of drugs. As Philip Hickey, PhD., puts it, "The stark reality is that **the individuals are being forcibly drugged into quietude** *[emphasis mine]*, and this is being done under the guise of providing 'treatment' for an 'illness.'"[57]

Once hospital personnel perceive that the immediate danger is gone, patients are sent back out into the world where the same stressors they had previously experienced will be encountered. All the support systems vanish overnight, which actually makes the return home a very dangerous time. Any anxieties, fears, distress, or other negative emotions felt before hospitalization often return. Now the patient may interpret the return of those pains *even after being treated in a hospital* as a sign that there is no help to be had and no hope for recovery or improvement.

Many researchers recognize that discharging patients into the same environment with the same stressors that existed before commitment poses a danger, especially since the patients think that "there was indeed no help and no connection, and they are still suffering unbearable psychic pain."[58] The danger is compounded by the fact that a person who has attempted suicide "to escape from an emotional crisis often develops a pattern in which suicide attempts occur in similar crises. For these people, a suicide attempt actually offers a temporary solution and, often, a sense of relief."[59]

Is there any hope? An emerging view in suicide research is that it is absolutely essential to establish individualized safety strategies so that patients can cope with emotional upheaval. One of the best ways to do this is with CBT (Cognitive Behavioral Therapy), which challenges patients' flawed patterns of thinking about the self and the world so that negative behaviors can be changed.

When used for patients who have attempted suicide, CBT focuses on enhancing coping skills, minimizing social isolation, increasing adherence to treatment, and implementing emergency safety plans.

One study indicates that nine hours of individual CBT for the prevention of suicide can reduce repeat suicide attempts in approximately 50 percent of patients. Sadly, the same study indicates that "only some [health-care practitioners] are knowledgeable about how to best use CBT with a suicidal patient."[60] Perhaps Evie could have been saved if her private therapist had been trained in CBT or in another action-oriented form of therapy called DBT.

Dialectical behavior therapy (DBT) combines cognitive-behavioral therapy (CBT) with humanistic elements and mindfulness, the practice of being fully aware of and present in the moment. It also involves teaching people how to tolerate distress rather than attempting to change it, and how to develop interpersonal effectiveness and regulate emotions.

According to researchers at the University of Washington, this therapeutic approach has "outperformed control treatments in reducing intentional self-injury, suicidal ideation, inpatient hospitalizations, hopelessness, depression, dissociation, anger, and impulsivity."[61]

Perhaps these behavioral therapy approaches work because they depend on the patient's active involvement, thereby giving the patient feelings of self-worth and competence.

Watching how patients were treated in Brunswick Hospital and learning about Evie's experiences with in- and out-patient treatment convinced me that prevention of repeated suicide attempts *must* start with investing patients with a belief that they and their lives have value.

The practices at Brunswick certainly didn't foster this belief. In fact, the practices in the hospital stripped patients of their dignity and denied them the right to participate in their treatment planning, or to even express concerns about their treatment. These practices made patients feel that they were incapable of managing their own lives and added to their feelings that their lives weren't worth very much.

Where were Brunswick's mental health professionals when the following psychological truism was being taught: "... all humans need to feel competent, autonomous, and related to others. Social contexts that facilitate satisfaction of these three basic psychological needs will support people's inherent activity, promote more optimal motivation, and yield the most positive psychological, developmental, and behavioural outcomes. In contrast, social environments that thwart satisfaction of these needs yield less optimal forms of motivation and have deleterious effects on a wide variety of well-being outcomes."[62]

Autonomy has long been recognized in psychology as a fundamental human need. In addition, there is a strong correlation between autonomy and motivation. "Research has shown that autonomous motivation predicts persistence and adherence and is advantageous for effective performance."[63]

Hospitalization or therapy that negates a suicidal patient's autonomy may very likely diminish the patient's motivation to get help. It is not, therefore, at all surprising that "having a follow-up appointment scheduled on discharge from either the emergency department or an inpatient service, whether or not it was actually kept ... significantly [reduced] the risk of dying on a subsequent attempt."[64] Moreover, the risk of a repeated suicide attempt has been shown to be significantly reduced when a person *keeps* scheduled follow-up appointments."[65]

It has been found that patients without an outpatient appointment after discharge are twice as likely to be re-hospitalized in the same year, and one study showed that when patients had a motivational interview prior to discharge, no-shows at the first outpatient appointment were significantly reduced.[66]

To reduce readmissions, the NYS Office of Mental Health has called for improved "engagement" in outpatient services. An article in *World Psychiatry: The Official Journal of the World Psychiatric Association* explains: "Poor engagement may lead to worse clinical outcomes, with symptom relapse and rehospitalization. … recovery-oriented care … prioritizes autonomy, empowerment and respect for the person receiving services … enhance engagement. … person-centered care, including shared decision making, is a treatment approach that focuses on an individual's unique goals and life circumstances."[67]

In spite of the clear correlation between repeat suicide attempts and patients' failure to receive additional treatment, more than 30 percent of people who had been hospitalized as the result of a suicide attempt were released without a follow-up appointment.[68]

The patients who voluntarily made follow-up appointments *wanted help and believed they could be helped.* No one forced or berated them into making those appointments; the patients merely followed suggestions or guidelines.

As one study of plans that are effective in reducing suicide recidivism put it, a "stay-in-contact" program "does not invade the daily life of suicidal attempters and can be employed in parallel to the eventual healthcare and offers a reliable and effective treatment in cases of suicidal crisis."[69] After hospitalization, a patient is in a sense "set adrift," and the sense of "connectedness" provided by active follow-up is critical.

The studies and data make it seem that hospitalization did little or nothing to give patients the tools they needed to *want* to live. The only reasons Evie could find to keep going were not hurting her family and friends and not abandoning her dog. For those on the edge of a decision to end their lives, those reasons are just not enough.

Wanting to live must begin with believing that one's life has value. To help patients find a way to go on living, hospitals must give patients a sense of their value by giving them respect and treating them with dignity. Hospitals must also give the patients some autonomy so that they learn to live in and deal with each moment that comes.

Dignity and respect can't be found in a pill.

Isolation from the world doesn't breed coping skills.

It's time for hospitals to turn to a new way of preventing repeated suicide attempts.

PART THREE

Alice tried another question.
"What sort of people live about here?"
In THAT direction," the Cat said,
waving its right paw round,
"lives a Hatter: And in THAT direction,"
waving the other paw, "lives a March Hare.
Visit either you like: they're both mad."
"But I don't want to go among mad people,"
Alice remarked.
"Oh, you can't help that," said the Cat:
"we're all mad here. I'm mad. You're mad."

Lewis Carroll

A Broken System

Mental health practices in the United States are not working. Alan and Evie were just two of the countless people who cannot find viable solutions to their difficulties.

Despite being in therapy and taking medications, despite being hospitalized twice because of suicide attempts and once because of a threat of suicide, Evie became one of the more than 38,000 people who take their own lives each year.

From the psychiatrists and psychologists who failed to diagnose Alan's PTSD to the physicians who wrote prescription after prescription to the social worker who didn't, couldn't, or wouldn't follow through on placing Alan in an appropriate program, the system is broken.

Among comparable countries, the U.S. has the highest rate of death from mental health and substance abuse — 12.0 per 100,000 population, compared to an average of 4.9 per 100,000 population in similarly wealthy countries.[70] Some might say the fault lies in an American society that has lost its core, a society that is too fragmented, leaving people feeling alienated, alone and adrift. This may be so, but a mental health system riddled with problems is not providing the help it should.

For the millions of Americans who suffer from schizophrenia or bipolar disorder, for those who can't get out of bed in the morning because of depression, for those who can't walk out the door of their homes because of anxiety, good mental health care is the only door to their leading fully functioning lives.

Yet, according to the Substance Abuse and Mental Health Services Administration, less than 40 percent of people with mental health issues receive the care they need due to stigma, limited availability of care, inadequate finances... the list goes on.

Access to care is limited

Tragically, scores of people who suffer from mental health issues are unable or unwilling to get professional help. Some do not seek treatment because of the weight of shame and the fear of stigma.

In a recent survey of people who recognized they needed help but weren't getting it, 15 percent cited their fear that others would find out and have a negative opinion. Another 7 percent were afraid of possible negative effects on their jobs and 5.9 percent were concerned about confidentiality in general.

Mentally ill people are all too aware that they are often seen as incompetent at best and dangerous at worst. Many of the mentally ill — especially those who suffer from depression—are all too often told to "snap out of it" as if they are responsible for or have made some kind of choice regarding their illness. When the mentally ill take these negative images to heart, the resulting loss of self-esteem may lead them to believe that they do not deserve treatment or that they can never recover.

"The prejudice and discrimination of mental illness is as disabling as the illness itself. It undermines people attaining their personal goals and dissuades them from pursuing effective treatments," says psychological scientist Patrick W. Corrigan of the Illinois Institute of Technology, lead author of a report published in *Psychological Science in the Public Interest.*[71]

Another factor limiting people's access to care is economic: The costs involved in mental health treatment are prohibitively high when insurance does not cover the majority of treatment. Cost is actually the most commonly reported structural barrier (as opposed to attitudinal barriers) to using mental health services.[72]

More than 50 percent of respondents to a 2011 survey said they couldn't afford mental health care whether or not they had health insurance;

15 percent of respondents said that their health insurance didn't cover it or didn't cover enough.[73]

Even after passage of the Affordable Care Act, more than 27 million Americans were uninsured and "high deductibles and out of pocket costs still remain the biggest barrier preventing individuals from seeking mental health treatment."[74]

The national average for therapy sessions is $75 to $150 per session; in New York, that average jumps to $200 to $300 per session.[75] Some estimates indicate that out-patient therapy sessions can amount to $120 to $1,200 in out-of-pocket costs each month.[75] Private psychiatric hospitals — and there aren't many of them—can cost $30,000 per month and some do not accept insurance.[76]

Medicaid is usually not an option as federal law prevents the government's paying for long-term institutional care. The cost of inpatient psychiatric hospitalization in public hospitals ranges from $2,900 to $13,300 for an average stay of eight days; only about 28 percent of these stays are covered by Medicaid.[77]

Because people cannot pay for outpatient treatment, they often head to emergency rooms in times of dire distress such as severe anxiety attacks, suicidal ideation, agitation that can't be calmed, or if they fear harming harming others.

Approximately five million people each year visit emergency rooms with mental disorders as the primary diagnosis.[78] Between 2001 and 2011, 6 percent of all emergency department patients had a psychiatric condition.[79] Because these mental health crises are not deemed life-threatening, patients visiting the ER for mental health issues are triaged to the back of the line. When there are many mentally distressed people to care for in addition to other patients, total waiting time for *all* patients who go to the ER increases.

Placement for the mentally ill after an ER visit is also a problem. There is a critical shortage of beds in state-run psychiatric hospitals. In 2016, there were roughly 37,680 state psychiatric beds available—only 11.7 beds per 100,000 population. Mental health advocates recommend 40 beds per 100,000 people, but the number of beds has been steadily declining due to budget cuts as well as a shortage of mental health professionals.[80]

Because of this, mentally ill patients with severe symptoms are being held in emergency rooms—some for weeks—during which time they receive little or no mental health care. This only compounds the overall wait time and quality-of-service issues that emergency rooms have come to be known for.[80]

In addition, the *Psychiatric Times* reports, "The pressure on existing beds [in hospitals] is so intense that patients are discharged prematurely [from emergency rooms] and often have to be readmitted or end up homeless or incarcerated."[81]

Some go so far as to say that prisons in the U.S. are "warehouses" for the severely mentally ill. A 2018 survey of community jails in Maryland, for instance, revealed that inmates who had a psychiatric illness but did not have a court order committing them had to wait an average of 87 days for treatment.[82]

Psychiatric Hospitals Offer Inadequate Care

Getting a bed in a psychiatric hospital is far from a guarantee of quality mental health care. Nowhere is the failure of mental health practices more apparent than in these institutions where budgetary concerns appear to outweigh the need for best practices. Another volume would be needed to review and examine the use of "best medical practices" in the nation's psychiatric hospitals.

My own personal experience at Brunswick Hospital is just one story among many thousands that provide evidence of this sad situation

One of the indications that psychiatric hospitals are "broken" is the disturbingly high rate of readmission for psychiatric patients—referred to as the "revolving door" phenomenon.[83] As the Healthcare Costs and Utilization Project (HCUP) puts it, "Hospital readmission within 30 days of discharge usually represents a negative clinical outcome for patients with mental disorders..."[84]

According to data from HCUP, 12.8 percent of mental disorder discharges and 9.9 percent of substance abuse related discharges are readmitted for the same type of diagnosis within 30 days. On the other hand, the readmission rate for hospitalized people who had no mental health or substance abuse conditions is only 4.8 percent.

It's no wonder a National Academy of Sciences report devotes an entire section to "Quality Problems Hinder Effective Treatment and Recovery" in mental health facilities.[85] The Medicare Payment Advisory Commission (MedPAC) also reported that hospital readmission may indicate poor care or, in some cases, missed opportunities to better coordinate care.[86]

Consider these statistics:

- 15 percent of patients with mood disorders are readmitted within 30 days[87]
- Behavioral health discharges ranked among the top five diagnostic categories for 30-day readmissions in 15 states[88]
- Between 40 to 50 % of psychiatric readmissions occur within 12 months of the original hospitalization[89]

The high rates of readmission aren't surprising considering that the Institute of Medicine reports numerous studies document a discrepancy between mental health care that is known to be effective and the care that is actually delivered.

A review of studies published from 1992 through 2000 assessing the quality of care for many different mental and substance abuse illnesses found that only 27 % of the studies reported adequate rates of adherence to established clinical practice guidelines. Later studies have continued to document departures from evidence-based practice guidelines."[90]

One of the practices at Brunswick that struck me as very questionable was the way that decisions about medications were made. At Brunswick, it seemed that choice of appropriate medications failed to take into account a basic premise of scientific inquiry. Students of high school science learn that controls are a very basic part of the scientific method. Without them, the results of an experiment cannot be considered reliable. In a controlled experiment, there is only one variable and the possibility of effects from other variables is minimized if not eliminated.

Hoping that meciation would alleviate my depression, the psychiatrist at Brunswick ordered two different medications on the first day of my stay. If there had been a change in my behavior or attitude, how could the psychiatrist have determined which of the psychiatric medications was responsible for producing that effect? Which pill was working? Was a combination of pills required? Which combination? How could anyone know which meds were having which effect?

What role did other non-psychiatric medications play in the observed effects? Furthermore, what objective measurements were used to determine efficacy? No brain scans, no blood tests, no cognitive tests were administered at Brunswick — are they administered elsewhere?

In Brunswick, as in other psychiatric hospitals and doctors' offices, patients were merely given a checklist of activities and feelings with questions such as "Are you sleeping more?" "Have you lost interest in activities you used to enjoy?"

From day to day, if not minute to minute, especially for someone under mental and emotional duress, responses to such questions will vary depending on a given day's circumstances. Treatments are chosen based on the patients' accounts of their feelings and activities.

Ironically, when such "anecdotal evidence" is presented in support of alternative, Eastern/Chinese, or other "alternative" medicine, it is routinely ridiculed and derided by establishment health-care professionals. And yet, in the mental health scene, anecdotal evidence is the standard method of judgement of efficacy.

In addition, I witnessed how the psychiatric hospital experience frequently strips people of dignity and any sense of responsibility or control over their lives. The hospital treats the patient like a child and says, "We know what you need." It in no way affords individuals the sense that they are worthwhile human beings with the right to happy, productive lives.

How can — and why would — patients who feel less than worthy put forth the effort to fight for their lives? And my experiences reveal the workings of just one psychiatric hospital. This same process likely plays out in psychiatric hospitals throughout the country.

Evidence supporting the claim that psychiatric hospitals are failing in their mission can be seen in readmission rates.

One can only imagine the pain, frustration and perhaps even despair of the patients and families caught in the revolving door of readmissions. We can, however, calculate the dollars and cents involved: In 2007, New York State estimated a cost of over $202 million for mental health readmissions.[91] Nationally, mood disorders and serious mental illnesses led to 77,400 readmissions and $588 million in additional costs.[92]

Additional Psychiatrists are Needed

Given the poor quality of inpatient psychiatric care, people who seek help for mental health conditions likely desire to avoid stays in psychiatric hospitals and prefer to look for outpatient treatment with a local psychiatrist.

Unfortunately, there is *also* a serious shortage of psychiatrists and mental health care professionals. This lack of trained mental health professionals makes it very difficult for those seeking help to actually get it.

The Health Resource and Services Administration (HRSA) considers an adequate number of psychiatrists to be about 3.3 psychiatrists per 100,000 population. Nationally, there are 13.5 psychiatrists per 100,000 population."[93] In 2017, New American Economy reported, "More than 60 percent of all counties in the United States—including 80 percent of all rural counties—do not have a single psychiatrist."[94]

In July 2017, the Henry J. Kaiser Family Foundation reported that for mental health, the population-to-provider ratio must be at least 30,000 to 1 (20,000 to 1 if there are unusually high needs in the community).[95] It is estimated that 111 million people are living in areas where there is a shortage of mental health professionals.[96]

Another Kaiser Family Foundation report reported that in December 2018, there were only enough practitioners to satisfy 26.10% of the need in the U.S.; an additional 6,894 practitioners were needed to fulfill that need. The number of additional practitioners needed is based on a population-to-psychiatrist ratio of 30,000 to 1 (20,000 to 1 where high needs are indicated).[97]

Alan's experiences are a grim testimony of the shortage. Toward the end of his life, he made repeated phone calls to psychiatrists and to intensive outpatient facilities. Time and again, he was met with the comment that no new patients could be seen.

Given the consequences of untreated mental illness and considering the number of people who suffer, it is surprising that the shortage is not being addressed.

In speaking to the American Psychiatric Association's 2014 annual meeting, then-Vice President Joseph Biden said the U.S. had a "desperate" need for more psychiatrists. According to *US News and World Report,* "Medical students choosing the field of psychiatry are fewer in number than in decades past. ...many graduates face huge debt burdens, and psychiatry is among the lowest-paid of the medical specialties (especially when working in clinics and public hospitals where they are needed the most)."[98]

Lawrence Kelmenson, M.D., who has practiced psychiatry for more than 30 years, discussed the problem in a 2017 issue of the online newsletter *Mad in America: Science, Psychiatry and Social Justice.* As he sees it, the profession of psychiatry fell into disrepute beginning in the early 1960s with Thomas Szasz's *The Myth of Mental Illness.* Szasz claimed that society used the term "mentally ill" to explain people's "irregularities." A bit later, Dr. Kelmenson points out, the Rosenhan Experiment indicated that mental health professionals could not reliably tell the difference between people who were sane and those who were insane.[99]

Subsequently, many medical students avoided a profession in which they would be considered hacks.

Around the same time, both state and private psychiatric hospitals began to close, forcing psychiatrists to move from inpatient to outpatient practice. The number of psychologists and social workers offering therapy to patients increased substantially, and their services were in demand because their fees were substantially less. This fierce competition in the field helped diminish doctors' motivation to continue their studies in order to practice psychiatry.

Insurance companies' policies further reduced motivation by curtailing the number of psychotherapy visits they would reimburse and requiring mountains of paperwork to prove the need for therapy.

The United States entered a new era with a very limited number of psychiatrists, and most of these are little more than "pill-pushers." It became far more lucrative for psychiatrists to just write prescriptions: They could then see four patients in an hour instead of spending one hour in analysis with a single patient.

Psychoanalysts — psychologists and social workers — have taken up the job of talk therapy instituted by Sigmund Freud and immortalized in W.H. Auden's poem "In Memory of Sigmund Freud":

> *He wasn't clever at all: he merely told*
> *the unhappy Present to recite the Past*
> *like a poetry lesson till sooner*
> *or later it faltered at the line where*
>
> *long ago the accusations had begun,*
> *and suddenly knew by whom it had been judged,*
> *how rich life had been and how silly,*
> *and was life-forgiven and more humble,*
>
> *able to approach the Future as a friend*
> *without a wardrobe of excuses, without*
> *a set mask of rectitude or an*
> *embarrassing over-familiar gesture...*

Training Is Inadequate

Increased numbers of beds and professionals alone won't repair the broken mental health system. Better training of mental health professionals is absolutely essential. Psychotherapy is certainly one of the major tools in the mental health system, and there is a great deal of evidence that it can be an effective treatment.

There is also evidence that a significant number of patients fail to improve with psychotherapy. One researcher points out that "30 percent of patients fail to respond during clinical trials, and as many as 65 percent of patients in routine care leave treatment without a measured benefit."[100] Another study indicated that 5-10 percent of the patients in its clinical trials completed treatment "worse off than before."[101]

Further evidence that training for psychotherapists needs reevaluation is the fact that patients often experience deterioration in their conditions. "...deterioration varied from a low of 3.2 percent to a high of 14 percent, with an average rate of 8 percent."[102]

One review of practices published in the *Annual Review of Clinical Psychology* discussed the need for clinicians to use "outcome measures" in their practice, saying, "Clinicians are encouraged to employ these methods in routine practice."[103]

Horst Kachele, M.D., Ph.D. and Joseph Schachter, M.D., Ph.D., point out that psychotherapy may have "side effects, destructive processes, and negative outcomes" and that therapists "are unfamiliar with methods and criteria for identifying and preventing negative outcomes."[104] Yet another study involving young adults' failure to improve with therapy looked at therapists who "seem not to have succeeded in adjusting their technique to their patients' core problems."[105]

With respect to suicide specifically, the American Association of Suicidology (AAS) reports that mental health professionals lack training in the critical arena of suicide-risk assessment. "We just know that so many psychologists, as well as other mental health professionals, are inadequately trained or not trained at all in suicide prevention, assessment and management," says William "Bill" Schmitz Jr., PsyD, president of the association and chair of its task force on suicide risk assessments. "...the neglect of this issue leaves psychologists ill-prepared to deal with the worst possible treatment outcome — death."

A large number of students in psychology graduate schools are trained only on suicide statistics and risk factors, not in clinical methods of conducting meaningful suicide risk assessments. AAS has asked that accrediting organizations, state licensing boards, and new state and federal legislation require suicide-specific training.[106]

Another at-risk group that mental health professionals may not be serving adequately is the LBGTQ (lesbian, bisexual, gay, transgender, queer) community.

The National Alliance on Mental Illness (NAMI) points out "Though more therapists and psychiatrists today have positive attitudes toward the LGBTQ community, people still face unequal care due to a lack of training and/or understanding. Health care providers still do not always have up-to-date knowledge of the unique needs of the LGBTQ community or training on LGBTQ mental health issues. Providers who lack knowledge and experience working with members of the LGBTQ community may focus more on a person's sexual orientation and/or gender identity than a person's mental health condition."[107]

As previously discussed, diagnosis and treatment of PTSD are other areas in which therapists seem to need more rigorous training. Today, trauma counseling certificate programs are *offered* to professionals to provide training in various PTSD treatment methods. Such certificates are not, however, required of mental health professionals.

A number of the certificate programs seem to emphasize therapeutic approaches for soldiers, which is long overdue. According to the Department of Veterans Affairs, in 2014 an average of 20 Veterans committed suicide each day, amounting to 18 % of all adult suicides, while Veterans constituted 8.5% of the U.S. population.[108]

The federal government is aware of the need for improved training. In its 2013 report to Congress, The Substance Abuse and Mental Health Services Administration (SAMHSA) reported that many professionals including social workers and psychologists are "likely to have insufficient training in behavioral health." The report also states, "SAMHSA is keenly aware that to achieve its mission to reduce the impact of substance abuse and mental illness on America's communities, a well-trained, educated and fully functioning workforce is needed."[109]

One of the agency's initiatives to accomplish this goal is the publication of TIPS: Treatment Improvement Protocols for best practice guidelines for the treatment of substance abuse. To create these TIPS, a panel of researchers, clinicians, program administrators, and patient advocates brings their expertise to the table to arrive at "a consensus on best practices." The findings are available on the Internet and are distributed to clinicians and program administrators.[110]

Another of SAMHSA's initiatives seeks to advance a recovery-oriented approach to mental health care in the belief that overcoming the challenges is the foundation of recovery.[111] SAMHSA recognizes that many health care professionals do little more than administer drugs to *lessen the severity of symptoms*: the absence of symptoms is *not* a return to a "normal" state of mind or of health.

If a patient takes pain-killers to relieve a toothache, does he recover from the cavity or abscess? If psychic pain is relieved by medication, is the patient recovering from the disease causing the pain?

When the Substance Abuse and Mental Health Services Administration says it is developing materials and programs to "foster a better understanding of recovery, recovery-oriented practices, and the roles of the various professions in promoting recovery" and will use those programs to "train thousands of psychiatrists, psychologists, psychiatric nurses, nurses, social workers and mental health peer specialists," it seems clear that the current cadre of mental health professionals has not been fully trained in helping patients recover.

Perhaps it is not surprising that many people rely on drugs and other substances to help them deal with their mental health problems.

Americans Depend on a "Magic Bullet"

Americans are drug-obsessed. Whether it is laziness, a lack of willpower, or a lack of work ethic, Americans seem to prefer a pound of curc (in pill form) over even an ounce of prevention.

Walk into the drug section of any supermarket or chain pharmacy today and you will see rows and rows of over-the-counter (OTC) medications, vitamins, and supplements. In one store alone, two sides of a ten-foot aisle are occupied by shelves filled with nothing but cough and cold medicines.

According to the Consumer Healthcare Products Association (CHPA), there are more than 100,000 OTC drug products on the market today. Obviously, medication is a big business. It is estimated that OTC sales alone in the United States reached around $34.3 billion U.S. dollars in 2017; in 1965 that number was $2 billion. Perhaps our obsession started when Alexander Fleming discovered penicillin in 1928.

By the 1940s, the active ingredient in Alexander Fleming's discovery had been isolated and penicillin began to be used to treat previously untreatable illnesses such as pneumonia, scarlet fever, diphtheria, and tuberculosis. "The age of healing miracles had come at last, wrote Louis Sutherland in his book *Magic Bullets*.[112]

So many people came to believe that penicillin was a magic bullet that they asked their doctors for prescriptions even when there was no evidence of a bacterial infection. And we all paid the price.

Today, drug-resistant bacteria are common. Penicillin is no longer recommended as the first treatment for Staphylococcus infections because it is effective in less than 10 percent of new cases, and the growing problem of antibiotic-resistant bacteria has compromised the efficacy of many other important antibiotics. Our reliance on anti-psychotic medications also comes with a cost.

In his 2010 book *Anatomy of an Epidemic,* Robert Whitaker suggests that our reliance on psychopharmacology is fueling an increase in mental illness. His contention is backed by numerous scientific studies in highly respected journals. Some of those studies indicate that people who use psychiatric medications over an extended period of time also may become more prone to physical illness. He speaks of "our societal delusion about a psychopharmacology revolution."[113]

Among the statistics Whitaker cites is the increase in Social Security benefits to people with mental illness. (Unfortunately, some of this increase may be the result of people's taking advantage of loopholes in disability requirements.) Less than one million people were receiving SSI and SSDI in 1987 due to mental illness; by 2013 that number had increased to 3,599,417.

John Horgan, director of the Center for Science Writings at the Stevens Institute of Technology, considered this issue in "Are Psychiatric Medications Making Us Sicker" in *The Chronicle of Higher Education*. He writes, "If Whitaker is right, American psychiatry, in collusion with the pharmaceutical industry, is perpetrating what may be the biggest case of iatrogenesis—harmful medical treatment—in history."

Horgan also provides evidence supporting Whitaker's supposition: "...over the past few decades the proportion of Americans diagnosed with mental illness has skyrocketed. ...This epidemic has coincided, paradoxically, with a surge in prescriptions for psychiatric drugs. Between 1985 and 2008, sales of antidepressants and antipsychotics multiplied almost fiftyfold, to $24.2-billion." Horgan also points out, "A multi-nation report by the World Health Organization in 1998 associated long-term antidepressant usage with a higher rather than a lower risk of long-term depression."[114]

In September 2017, a study conducted by Jeffrey Vittengl at Truman University and published in *Psychotherapy and Psychosomatics* indicated that patients who had taken antidepressants for nine years displayed more severe depression symptoms.[115]

A 2019 study in the same journal called for increased attention to "affective disturbances caused by medical drugs" used in mental health treatment. These disturbances to moods, feelings, and attitudes are considered "iatrogenic," meaning that they are related to the treatment itself.

According to the authors of the article, "Affective disturbances caused by medical drugs, as well as paradoxical effects, manifestations of tolerance (loss of clinical effect, refractoriness), withdrawal and post-withdrawal disorders, are increasingly common due to the widespread use of psychotropic drugs in the general population. Such neglect is serious, since manifestations of behavioral toxicity are unlikely to respond to standard psychiatric treatments and may be responsible for the wide spectrum of disturbances subsumed under the generic rubric of treatment resistance."[116]

The dangers of worsening symptoms appear to be only the tip of the iceberg. In 2017, researchers at a public research university in Canada reviewed studies involving hundreds of thousands of people and reported that antidepressant users have a 14 percent higher risk of cardiovascular events such as strokes and heart attacks and a 33 percent higher chance of death than non-users.[117]

Many antidepressants work by blocking the absorption of serotonin by neurons. However, the heart, kidneys, lungs, and liver all use serotonin, too, and the antidepressants can interfere with the absorption of serotonin in these organs. The researchers warn that antidepressants could increase the risk of death by preventing various organs from functioning properly.

On the other hand, the researchers found that antidepressants do not have the same risk for those who *have* cardiovascular diseases, probably because the antidepressants have blood-thinning effects that are useful in treating such disorders. Furthermore, a study published in the *Annals of Medicine* in August 2018, concluded that there is evidence that "depression and antidepressant use may be associated with venous thromboembolism (VTE) risk, but the evidence is conflicting."[118]

With all of this information at hand, it is not surprising that Lawrence Kelmenson, MD, a practicing psychiatrist for 32 years, says, *Mad in America, June 9, 2019* "Psychiatrists are seen as hard-working, caring, understanding healers, but they're really snake-oil salesmen, drug-dealers, and master-sedaters. What they do should be illegal. Someday everyone will realize that not only do psychiatrists not heal anything, they're a major contributor to the recent rise in suicides and overdoses."[11]

Furthermore, The National Center for Health Research published an article entitled "Do Antidepressants Increase Suicide Attempts? Do They

Have Other Risks?" in which the authors state that antidepressants "have risks that outweigh the benefits for more patients than you probably realize."[120] One of these risks is suicide, which the article concludes is an unresolved controversy.

However, the article goes on to cite studies indicating an increase in violent behavior among those using Selective serotonin reuptake inhibitor (SSRIs) and reports that the FDA has issued a warning on all antidepressants administered to children and adults.

A study of 27,000 women conducted by the Centers for Disease Control and Prevention (CDC) reported that Paxil (paroxetine) and Prozac (fluoxetine) taken by pregnant women increase the risks for heart and neurological defects in newborn babies by as much as 3.5 times.

Seroquel (quetiapine) and Abilify (aripiprazole), usually prescribed as antipsychotics, are sometimes used to treat depression when other drugs have proven ineffective, and carry such risks as dramatic weight gain and "sudden cardiac death." The article also reports that "women taking SSRIs are more than 50% more likely to have a bone fracture."

Since the dangers seem real, why have prescriptions for antidepressants and other psychoactive medications increased so much?

It all started with chlorpromazine, which was synthesized in December 1951 in laboratories in France. The drug shortly became available by prescription and revolutionized the treatment of mental health. Gone were institutions like the infamous Bedlam in London; gone were lobotomies; soon electroshock vanished as well.

In 1952, Smith Kline purchased the rights to chlorpromazine and began marketing it as an anti-vomiting treatment while the company attempted to convince psychology departments and medical schools to test the drug as a treatment for mental illness. Eventually, Smith Kline convinced state governments that use of the drug would save them money since its use would decrease the number of patients in mental institutions. In 1954, Thorazine received FDA approval and psychopharmacology was born.

The pharmaceutical industry soon recognized that psychiatry could be the goose that lay the golden egg and began to court psychiatrists and their professional organizations. In addition to a stream of free gifts and meals, drug companies offered hefty pay to psychiatrists to be consultants and speakers, and subsidized various professional conferences. When some states passed laws requiring drug companies to report these payments to doctors, it was revealed that psychiatrists received more money than physicians in any other specialty.[121]

One of the leaders of modern psychiatry, Leon Eisenberg, a professor at Johns Hopkins and then Harvard Medical School, eventually voiced strong opposition to the use of drugs—a use he felt was advanced by the pharmaceutical industry.

Marcia Angell, M.D., goes even further in expressing doubts about the prescribing of drugs for mental illness. A former editor of *The New England Journal of Medicine* and currently a member of the faculty of the Department of Global Health and Social Medicine at Harvard Medical School, Dr. Angell writes in "The Illusions of Psychiatry," "Unlike the conditions treated in most other branches of medicine, there are no objective signs or tests for mental illness—no lab data or MRI findings—and the boundaries between normal and abnormal are often unclear. That makes it possible to expand diagnostic boundaries or even create new diagnoses... And drug companies have every interest in inducing psychiatrists to do just that... "[122]

Negative side effects aren't the only drawback to antidepressant use. There is also a considerable body of evidence that antidepressants are not very effective.

In 2013, authors of an article in *The Journal of the American Medical Association* reviewed 30 years of data and concluded that the effects of antidepressants were "nonexistent-to-negligible among depressed patients with mild, moderate, and severe baseline symptoms, whereas they were large for patients with very-severe symptoms."[123]

In 2015, an article in the journal of the world psychiatric association pointed out, "Simple biochemical theories that link low levels of serotonin with depressed mood are no longer tenable."[124] In addition, Whitaker says, "For the past twenty-five years, the psychiatric establishment has told us a false story. It told us that schizophrenia, depression, and bipolar illness are known to be brain diseases, even though... it can't direct us to any scientific studies that document this claim. It told us that psychiatric medications fix chemical imbalances in the brain, even though decades of research failed to corroborate this."[125]

According to an NIH report, approximately 40 to 60 out of 100 people taking antidepressants notice an improvement in six to eight weeks. However, in the same time period, 20 to 40 out of 100 taking a placebo notice improvement in symptoms.[126] A 2017 study of data from almost 7,000 patients published in the prestigious *Journal of the American Medical Association (JAMA)* has now shown that antidepressants are more effective than placebos, *but* the difference is minor and varies according to the type of mental disorder.[127]

This 2017 study published in the journal *JAMA Psychiatry* revealed that the placebo effect played a significant role in the efficacy of antidepressants. It also found that patients treated with antidepressants complained of greater side effects than those who received a placebo. The side effects ranged from mild symptoms such as headaches to suicidal behavior.

The study concluded, "There is some evidence for the benefit of selective serotonin reuptake inhibitors and serotonin-norepinephrine reuptake inhibitors in children and adolescents, but owing to the higher risk for severe adverse events, a cautious and individual cost-benefit analysis is of importance."[127]

Despite these studies, and largely because of the influence of the pharmaceutical, advertising and healthcare industries, antidepressants are the most commonly prescribed form of drug with approximately one in ten Americans taking antidepressants.

In 2005, PLOS Medicine, a peer-reviewed weekly medical journal, claimed that direct-to-consumer (DTC) advertising of selective serotonin reuptake inhibitor (SSRI) antidepressants has been "highly successful. ...

For instance, sertraline (Zoloft) was the sixth best-selling medication in the US in 2004, with over $3 billion in sales likely due, at least in part, to the widely disseminated advertising campaign starring Zoloft's miserably depressed ovoid creature. Research has demonstrated that class-wide SSRI advertising has expanded the size of the antidepressant market, and SSRIs are now among the best-selling drugs in medical practice."[128]

Another study found that "Patients' requests have a profound effect on physician prescribing in major depression and adjustment disorder" and concluded that DTC advertising has the potential to promote overuse.[129] The article also claims that "These advertisements present a seductive concept, and the fact that patients are now presenting with a self-described 'chemical imbalance' shows that the DTCA is having its intended effect: the medical marketplace is being shaped in a way that is advantageous to the pharmaceutical companies."

David Mischoulon, M.D., Ph.D., associate professor of psychiatry at Harvard Medical School and director of research at Massachusetts General Hospital's Depression and Clinical Research Program, was quoted by Web MD as saying, "We have known for many, many years that these antidepressants don't have the kinds of response rates in the real world of practice that they have in clinical trials..." Dr. Mischoulon attributes this to the rigorous selection process involved in choosing subjects for the trials.[130]

Is it any wonder that Dr. Angell urges that Americans stop believing that psychoactive drugs are the best treatment for mental illness or emotional distress. "Both psychotherapy and exercise have been shown to be as effective as drugs for depression, and their effects are longer-lasting, but unfortunately, there is no industry to push these."[131] Nonetheless, these "alternative treatments" are receiving increasing attention.

"Anti Antidepressants" Offer Hope

In August 2017, *Time* magazine's cover proclaimed, "The *Anti* Antidepressant: Depression afflicts 16 million Americans. One-third don't respond to treatment."

The article referred to on the cover, "New Hope for Depression" includes descriptions of five "Drug-free treatments backed by science." The first of these is exercise, referred to as "one of the most-studied natural approaches to treating depression."[132]

Moreover, an article in the official journal of the Association of Medicine and Psychiatry reports, "Many studies have examined the efficacy of exercise to reduce symptoms of depression, and the overwhelming majority of these studies have described a positive benefit associated with exercise involvement ... Research also suggests that the benefits of exercise involvement may be long lasting."[133]

In fact, a report published in the *Journal of Psychiatric Research* examines 25 different studies and concludes that "regular exercise has a large and significant antidepressant effect in people diagnosed with moderate and severe depression." The authors of the research study believe, "Previous meta-analyses may have underestimated the benefits of exercise due to publication bias. Our data strongly support the claim that exercise is an evidence-based treatment for depression."[134]

In a subsequent study published in the same journal, 33,908 healthy participants were assessed for anxiety and depression over an 11-year period. It was shown that even one hour a week of regular exercise can protect against depression. People who did not engage in any exercise were 44% more likely to suffer from depression than people who exercised for one to two hours per week. Although exercising for just one hour per week could have prevented 12% of depression cases, it had no effect on anxiety.[135]

Furthermore, a study published in the American College of Sports Medicine's *Health Fit Journal* concluded that "exercise appears to be an effective treatment for depression, improving depressive symptoms to a comparable extent as pharmacotherapy and psychotherapy."[136]

The *Time* article's list of effective non-drug treatments for depression also includes various "talk therapies" that are vastly different from hours of analysis. One of these is cognitive-behavioral therapy (CBT), which emphasizes changing negative thought patterns. Patients learn that they can take control of the way they interpret things in their environment.

Another kind of talk therapy that has scientific backing for its effectiveness is behavioral-activation therapy, which aims to alleviate the withdrawal from life that characterizes depression. Patients learn to identify their negative behavior patterns and then to choose behaviors that are positive replacements. These positive behaviors are easy to implement and are rewarding—reading, volunteering, being with friends.

Another successful type of talk therapy listed in *Time* is mindfulness-based cognitive therapy (MBCT) training. In April 2016, Reuters Health reported on a study conducted in the United Kingdom that analyzed data on 1,258 people who had participated in nine randomized controlled trials. These trials compared MBCT to other treatments for recurring depression. People receiving MBCT were found to be about 31 percent less likely to have depression again after 60 weeks in comparison to people who received other treatments, including self-help.[137]

The last on *Time*'s list of non-drug treatments is transcranial magnetic stimulation. In this noninvasive procedure, a large magnetic coil is held on a person's head. Small electric currents are passed through the coil which then creates magnetic fields. These fields stimulate nerve cells in the area of the brain believed to be involved in mood. The effects are significant enough that the procedure was approved by the FDA for treatment of depression in those who haven't responded to at least one antidepressant.

Perhaps the mental health industry will begin to choose non-invasive and non-pharmaceutical treatments as the first choice in treatment.

Although the *Time* article does not mention diet, there is a large and growing body of evidence linking diet and depression. One of the nutrients touted for its benefits in alleviating depression is tryptophan, which is found in turkey, seeds, nuts, eggs and dairy products.

This amino acid along with the B vitamins helps produce the mood-elevating chemical serotonin. A study published in *Acta Neuropsychiatrica* in 2011 concluded that changing a person's level of tryptophan may be beneficial if there is a "personal or family history of depression."[138]

Low vitamin B_{12} and low folate have been found in studies of depressed patients, and an association between depression and low levels of these two vitamins is found in studies of the general population as reported in *Journal of Psychopharmacology* in 2005.[139] Several studies since then have confirmed the association.

In 2010, two researchers reported in *Alternative Medicine Review,* "Supplementation with folate may help reduce depressive symptoms." The researchers point out that folate is necessary for the synthesis of norepinephrine, serotonin, and dopamine."[140]

In the same year, in a study of 3,503 adults aged 65 and up, higher total intakes of vitamins B-6 and B-12 "were associated with a decreased likelihood of incident depression for up to 12 y[ears] of follow-up."[141] Vegan and vegetarian diets are notoriously low in B-vitamins, and an article by Daniel Rosenfeld of Cornell University published in 2018 stated that vegetarians are more likely to be depressed than meat-eaters.[142] On the other hand, consuming foods rich in Omega-3 fatty acids may help alleviate depression. These fatty acids play a critical role in the development and function of the central nervous system.

A meta-analysis of 31 studies involving more than 20,000 cases of depression was published in the *Journal of Affective Disorders* in 2016 and supported the claim that dietary omega-3 is associated with a lower risk of depression.[143]

Moreover, a growing body of evidence indicates that the organisms which live in our gastrointestinal tracts (commonly referred to as the *gut microbiome* or *gut microbiota*) play an important but little understood role in mental health. The evidence is so strong that in 2015 the National Institute of Mental Health awarded four grants worth up to $1 million each for research on the gut microbiome's role in mental disorders.

In that same year, an article in *Clinical Psychopharmacology and Neuroscience* called the gut-brain axis "the missing link in depression. In August 2017, Juan M. Lima-Ojeda, a physician and researcher at the University of Regensburg, Germany, reported "...there is strong communication between the gastrointestinal tract and the brain...changes to the microbiome-gut-brain axis could be associated with the etiology of different neuropsychiatric disorders such as depression."[144]

Mitchell L. Gaynor M.D., reports that "neurochemicals made by gut bacteria play a role in mood and other neurologic functions. So balancing gut bacteria through the consumption of probiotics such as *Lactobaccilli* and *Bifidobacteria* helps to elevate mood."[145]

In February 2019, results from the Flemish Gut Flora Project provided "population-scale evidence for microbiome links to mental health…"[146] The study revealed two bacterium that are associated with "higher quality of life indicators" — *F*aecalibacterium and Coprococcus bacteria — and two — *Dialister, Coprococcus spp.* which were "depleted in depression.[147]

Our over-reliance on antibiotics is a major contributing factor to changes in or even destruction of the gut microbiome. In seeking evidence about the relationship between antibiotics, the gut microbiome and depression, health records of more than one million people in Great Britain were studied. The researchers concluded that even one course of antibiotics can "significantly raise the risk of depression."[148]

In addition to antibiotics, bottle feeding and delivering babies by caesarean section (C-section) have also been implicated in development of mental health conditions. When the baby passes through the birth canal naturally, it is one of the first moments during which the baby is exposed to the un-sterile environment of the world. This is also the moment when baby's gut microbiome begins to be established.[149]

Obstetricians and certain hospital systems have become all too willing to perform caesarean section (C-section) procedures on birthing mothers; elective C-section rates have reached 30 percent in the U.S. and are even higher in other developed countries.

The process of breastfeeding continues to help baby grow its gut microbiome,[150] but mothers all too frequently eschew breastfeeding.

If the gut microbiome is even partially responsible for helping to produce the neurochemicals that regulate depression, shouldn't we be more concerned that we aren't affording newborns the chance to establish their intestinal flora? And how can we be surprised that so many young people are being prescribed antidepressants?

You aren't likely to see a television or magazine advertisement for breastfeeding, CBT, or transcranial magnetic stimulation any time soon, but you probably encounter several pharmaceutical antidepressant advertisements weekly.

As physician and drug addiction expert Gabor Mate says, "The dominant medical tendency in the past few decades has been to reduce mental illness to chemical imbalances in the brain—for example, a deficiency of the chemical messenger serotonin. The obvious solution is a drug to increase serotonin levels." Dr. Mate believes that these "biochemical explanations are dangerous oversimplifications.

The level, balance and activity of serotonin and other brain chemicals are, throughout a person's lifetime, affected by emotional stresses. Whether in our jobs or in our personal relationships, our interactions with the environment do much to determine our brain's chemistry."[151] Yet thousands upon thousands continue to believe that treating mental illness requires the use of medications.

"Magic Bullet" Turns Deadly

Americans' belief in the power of the pill and in the existence of a "magic bullet" may be contributing to the high number of fatal drug overdoses. Tragically, an estimated 70,200 people died of drug overdoses in 2017, making drug overdose the leading cause of accidental death in the U.S. More than 30 percent of these fatal overdoses involved a combination of benzodiazepines and opioids.[152]

The opioid "epidemic" may not seem to be related to the broken mental health system, however, substance dependence is a mental health issue. It is one of the diagnoses in the *Diagnostic and Statistical Manual of Mental Disorders* (DSM) where it is defined as "a maladaptive pattern of substance use leading to clinically significant impairment or distress."[153]

Not only is a substance use disorder (SUD) considered a mental illness, but addiction frequently exists side by side with other mental illnesses. In fact, approximately half of those with a mental disorder will also experience a substance use disorder, and roughly 60 percent of adolescents in community-based SUD treatment programs meet the diagnostic criteria for another mental illness.[154]

This simultaneous occurrence of two chronic conditions is known as "comorbidity." Results of a National Epidemiologic Survey on Alcohol and Related Conditions indicate that "The comorbidity between specific mood and anxiety disorders and specific drug use disorders is pervasive in the U.S. population."[155]

At a symposium on the topic of comorbidity of substance abuse and mental illnesses, Dr. Edward Nunes, a professor of psychiatry from Columbia University School of Medicine, noted that in those dependent on opiates, "rates of lifetime affective disorder (primarily depressive disorders) range from 16 percent to 75 percent." At the same symposium, Dr. Kathleen Brady of the Department of Psychiatry and Behavioral Sciences at the Medical University of South Carolina, reported, "PTSD is one of the most common anxiety disorders in individuals with substance use disorders."[156]

Patients in the study of more than 422,000 veterans who received opioids found that those who were also prescribed benzodiazepines were more likely to have been diagnosed with a psychiatric disorder, including post-traumatic stress disorder, other anxiety disorders, depression, and bipolar or psychotic disorders.

Many of the mental illnesses that appear as comorbid with SUD are routinely treated with benzodiazepines. Drugs such as Xanax, Valium, and Klonopin are typically used to treat anxiety, panic attacks, insomnia, and depression and can slow breathing, particularly when taken with alcohol or narcotics such as opioids.

Despite this danger, approximately 17 percent of people were prescribed both classes of drug at the same time.[157] In a five-year study of veterans, it was found that "About half of the deaths from drug overdose occurred when veterans were concurrently prescribed benzodiazepines and opioids."[158]

My son's lethal overdose was also caused by a combination of benzodiazepines for depression and anxiety along with an opioid pain-killer.

The National Institute on Drug Abuse has reported that when taken in combination with painkillers or narcotics, benzodiazepines can increase the likelihood of a fatal overdose as much as tenfold.

"What we're seeing is just like what happened with opioids in the 1990s,"said Anna Lembke, MD, chief of addiction medicine at Stanford University School of Medicine and author of *Drug Dealer, M.D.* "It really does begin with overprescribing. Liberal therapeutic use of drugs in a medical setting tends to normalize their use. People start to think they're safe and, because they make them feel good, it doesn't matter where they get them or how many they use."[159]

The dangers of the simultaneous prescriptions are substantiated by researchers at Stanford University School of Medicine who found that people who took both opioids and benzodiazepines had more than double the risk of those who took only opioids. They conclude that "if doctors stopped prescribing the drugs concurrently, there would be at least a 15 percent reduction in overdoses requiring hospitalization, whether the patients use opioids long term or occasionally."[160]

No wonder that in August 2016, the U.S. Food and Drug Administration released a "black box" warning—a warning of life-threatening risk —against taking both kinds of drugs together.

Back-alley drug dealers are not the major villains in the drama of drugs and death. "The prescription drug epidemic is first and foremost an epidemic of overprescribing," wrote Dr. Lembke in *Drug Dealer, M.D.*[161] Dr. Lembke goes on to say, "Of those who became addicts, 25 percent started with a prescription medication." Further evidence of physicians' complicity can be seen in the fact that prescription opioids were to blame in more than 35 percent of all opioid overdose deaths in 2017.[162]

At first glance, some statistics would seem to contradict Dr. Lembke's assertion. Between 2006 and 2010 the opioid overdose rate among those prescribed the drug was almost identical to the death rate among those who used the drug illicitly. Since 2016, the death rate for prescription drugs decreased while the death rate for users of fentanyl and heroin in the illicit market increased.

These statistics do not take into account the number of addicted patients who could no longer get their prescriptions and turned to street drugs. In fact, the Center for Disease Control and Prevention (CDC), reports that "Drug overdose deaths involving prescription opioids rose from 3,442 in 1999 to 17,029 in 2017."[163]

Dr. Marc Siegel, a professor of medicine and medical director of Doctor Radio at NYU Langone Medical Center concurs with Dr. Lembke: "The biggest culprits in this addiction epidemic are physicians."[164]

But it wasn't the physicians who lit the fire of opioid addiction: in an attempt to fill its coffers, "Big Pharma" ignited the spark.

In an interview on MSNBC On March 10, 2017, Dr. Lembke blamed the pharmaceutical industry for promoting the "myth" that people who received opiates for pain would not become addicted. Instead, these companies "created a nation of people who are addicted to opioids."

According to Dr. Lembke, physicians from the 1980s to the early 2000s were encouraged to prescribe opioids. This encouragement started slowly in the 1950s when pain management became a separate discipline, driven by the availability of opioids in the marketplace and by the pharmaceutical companies eager to make money from the sale of these drugs. The push to use opioids increased as the population aged and as people began to live longer with chronic illnesses and, therefore, had legitimate need for pain relief.

As Dr. Lembke explains, pharmaceutical companies initially offered doctors the same perks to dispense opioids as they had for them to dispense psychoactive drugs. Eventually, the practice was outlawed, and the pharmaceutical companies turned their attention to academic researchers and medical societies. Subsequently—and probably not coincidentally — medical societies for pain specialists began arguing for more liberal use of opioids to treat pain; the meds were presented as non-addicting.

A number of public health experts single out a letter to the editor in the *New England Journal of Medicine* in 1980 as the start of the crisis of over prescription. In the letter, Jane Porter and Dr. Hershel Jick of Boston University wrote that of their 11,000-plus patients treated with narcotics, there were only four cases of addiction. The letter is often referred to as evidence that long-term use of narcotics for pain is not addictive.

Indeed, a report in *The New England Journal of Medicine* in June 2017 revealed that the letter had been cited 608 times in 439 articles (72.2%) citing it as evidence that "addiction was rare in patients treated with opioids."[165] The authors of the letter, which included three M.D./Ph.Ds, concluded, "We believe that this citation pattern contributed to the North American opioid crisis by helping to shape a narrative that allayed prescribers' concerns about the risk of addiction associated with long-term opioid therapy."

With statistical corroboration in hand, it is understandable that physicians could be swayed by the pharmaceutical companies. When the American Pain Society began to promote pain as a "vital sign" in addition to pulse, breathing, blood pressure, and temperature, Purdue Pharma was one of 28 corporate donors to the "Partners Against Pain Campaign."[166]

And the pharmaceutical companies went even further: Purdue Pharma in 1998 distributed 15,000 copies of a video promoting the use of opioids. In this video —"I Got My Life Back" —a physician said that opioids "do not have serious medical side effects" and "should be used much more than they are."[167] Purdue also offered new patients a free first OxyContin prescription. In 2007, Purdue executives pleaded guilty to misbranding OxyContin as less addictive than it is.

Purdue Pharma was not alone in pushing opioids. Following the precedent set by the lawsuits filed against tobacco companies in the 1990s, 24 states have filed suit against pharmaceutical companies that had downplayed the addictive nature of the drugs. Ohio Attorney General Mike DeWine accused the companies' of spending millions on marketing campaigns that "falsely deny or trivialize the risks of opioids while overstating the benefits of using them for chronic pain."[168] On August 26, 2019, The New York Times reported that an Oklahoma judge had ruled that Johnson & Johnson "intentionally played down the dangers and oversold the benefits of opioids." The judge's ruling ordered the company to pay the state $572 million and called the company's marketing campaigns "false, misleading, and dangerous."

In addition, approximately 30 states have now instituted policies to set limits on the prescribing of opioids. With these policies in effect, opioid prescriptions decreased from a peak of more than 255 million in 2012 to 191 million in 2017.[169]

Even with the reduction in opioid prescriptions, approximately two million Americans are misusing prescription opioids and heroin.[170] As we have seen, many of these people are also suffering from a mental illness. Treating the addiction alone will not get to the root of the problem, which means that relapse is very likely to occur.

As a matter of fact,the National Institute on Drug Abuse has determined that "Treatment for comorbid illnesses should focus on both mental illness and substance use disorders together, rather than one or the other."[171]

Sadly, the social worker who recommended a drug treatment program for Alan apparently didn't know this. Even if she had, treatment might not have been available for him.

People on Medicaid, as Alan was, along with the thousands of uninsured have long waits to get into treatment facilities. For this reason, Michael Massing, author of a critique on the war against drugs, refers to the need for "repairing and expanding a treatment network that is severely underfunded, badly splintered and completely overwhelmed" as "the real scandal in the fight against opioids."[172]

In 2017, an estimated 19 percent of those who needed treatment actually received it. Those who do get treatment usually have private insurance and have access to treatment in facilities that can cost $10,000 a week.

Privacy Laws Protect Patients but Punish Families

Trying to help a child who is suffering from crippling psychic pain is a frustrating, emotionally draining and sometimes terrifying task. The problems are seriously compounded when that child turns 18 and becomes an "adult" in the eyes of the law.

In 1966, The Health Insurance Portability and Accountability Act (HIPAA) was created, in part, to ensure privacy and confidentiality of health records. As a result, once a child turns 18, a parent will be denied any information about a child's physical or mental condition unless the child consents —even if the parent is paying the bills.

Although the Privacy Rule's requirements are designed to be flexible enough to accommodate various circumstances, health care providers are silenced by their fear of expensive lawsuits. According to Jane Hyatt Thorpe, an associate professor at George Washington University's department of health policy and an expert on patient privacy, providers are often uncertain about the information they can legally share, so they just say "no," which they see as the safest course of action.[173] This is a dilemma for parents whose children are suffering from mental illness and may even be a danger for those children.

Mental Illness Policy.org has published a list of what it calls HIPAA "handcuffs."[174] Two of these include:

- When a mentally ill child (over 18) goes missing, families can do nothing to find him or her because hospitals and shelters can't tell the parents that the child is missing in the first place.
- When a child is prescribed medication or a follow-up appointment is scheduled, the parents can't be told, so they cannot help ensure the child's compliance.

According to Dr. E. Fuller Torrey, a psychiatrist and founder of Treatment Advocacy Center, sharing information with the family can be "crucial to a patient's care, helping to ensure that they stick with a treatment plan."[175]

One of the psychiatrists who was treating Alan told me he could not discuss Alan's case with me, but he sympathized because he knew that I was paying the bills. When I reached out to him, it was in the belief that he should have information about Alan's life history and behavior that Alan might not remember or be willing to share. Wouldn't a patient's interaction with family be useful to a mental health practitioner?

Too strict an adherence to HIPAA might be considered partially responsible for the shooting deaths of 32 people at Virginia Tech in April 2007. Because of the law, the mental health professionals who treated Seung Hui Cho before the shooting did not, and could not, legally communicate with his parents.

If they had, they would have learned of his extensive history of mental illness. Without that information, they assumed that his aberrant behavior at the time was a recent, temporary and perhaps non-serious occurrence.

Cho's parents said that if they had known what was going on at the college, they would have brought Seung Hui to treatment. Because no one, including their son, was reporting any problems, the parents assumed Cho had recovered and was doing fine. In fact, there is nothing in HIPAA that prevents providers from receiving info *from* family members, but staff at Seung Hui's college either didn't know this or were fearful of repercussions.

As with many laws, HIPAA was instituted with every good intention of protecting private information, an issue that has become even more important now in the Internet age. None of us should have to worry that marketers will obtain info they can use to hound us with sales pitches. More importantly, we should not have to worry that employers will have access to information that might give them a reason to dismiss us.

Denying parents access to information about their offspring is another issue. National Public Radio (NPR) reported the frustration of a parent whose son was hospitalized for the hallucinations, mania, and depression associated with schizophrenia.

When their son refused to give permission for his parents to speak with the doctors, the father said, "That was the first time we started feeling hopeless. ...Why am I as the one who is a primary care- giver, protector, provider, whatever—I've watched this kid grow up, and yet I'm out of the circle? I can't be there to be of help."[176]

In 2013, Timothy Murphy, a psychologist serving the 15th district of Pennsylvania, proposed the Helping Families in Mental Health Crisis Act, which was passed in an amended version in 2016.[177]

This amended version did not really ease health care providers' ability to share mental health information with families or caregivers. Although a section called "Compassionate Communication on HIPAA" was included, the bill turned the final decision on privacy over to the Department of Health and Human Services (HHS). The act says, " After finalizing regulations on the confidentiality of alcohol and drug abuse patient records, HHS must convene stakeholders to determine the effect of the regulations on patient care, health outcomes, and patient privacy."

The act also calls for HHS to "promulgate regulations clarifying the circumstances under which an entity may disclose protected health information" and to develop training programs for health care providers, legal professionals, patients and their families regarding protection and disclosure of health information for those with mental illnesses.

As a result, Health and Human Services published pages and pages of explication of HIPAA, the bottom line of which is, "HIPAA helps you stay connected with your loved one by permitting health professionals to contact you with information related to your family member, friend, or the person you are caring for, that is necessary and relevant to your involvement with the patient's health care or payment for care."[177]

However, because determining what is "necessary and relevant," is a subjective decision, the problems or "handcuffs" remain more on the shoulders' of health care providers than on HIPAA itself.

Health care providers don't necessarily understand the law; they are not legal experts and are fearful of law suits. Some health care providers may use the law to avoid having to deal with family members. Mental health practitioners need to realize that sharing information gives families the tools to ensure that patients arrive at counseling sessions and take their medications as prescribed.

Perhaps the law needs some tweaking, but it is definitely necessary for all health care providers to receive adequate training to ensure that HIPAA provisions are applied without harming those it was designed to protect.

Other solutions suggested by Mental Illness Policy.org include having HIPAA regulations that are clear enough so that it isn't necessary to hire a lawyer to understand them. The organization also recommends what it refers to as "safe harbor provisions," which "should insulate a person or organization from liability (or loss of funding) for making a disclosure with a good faith belief that the disclosure was necessary to protect the health, safety, or welfare of the person involved or members of the general public."[178]

Dr. Torrey also points out that the problem is HIPAA wasn't written with mental illness in mind. "When someone has cancer, you can make the assumption that their brain is working normally so that they can make an informed decision as to whether or not they want their loved ones to know exactly what the details of the cancer is. You can't make that assumption about people with schizophrenia or bipolar disorder."[179]

We also can't make that assumption about our offspring. Our children's decision to deny us the ability to discuss issues with mental health providers is more likely to be informed by anger, shame, guilt. or just plain adolescent rebelliousness than by rational judgement. Alan's decision not to allow the psychiatrist to talk to me was probably the result of all four.

As Alan got older and his need to be independent made him increasingly angry at me, he continued to deny me access to information from providers. At the same time, his depression, anxiety, and use of drugs were increasing. Phone calls I made to try to get him into rehab programs were always answered with, "We cannot talk to you. He has to make the call." The only way I could have had input was to go to court in order to have him declared unfit. At the time, that measure seemed far too extreme.

How devastating would it have been for a young man already scarred by lack of confidence to be declared unfit to take care of himself? Would he have been able to recover from such a blow to his fragile ego? If I'd had any inkling of where his problems would take him, I would, of course, have gone that route. In Alan's case, HIPAA was just one more indication of how broken the mental health care system is.

CONCLUSION

Flawed legislation... lack of access to mental health providers... debatable effectiveness of treatments... budgetary concerns taking precedence over best practices... over prescription of sometimes dangerous drugs... By itself, each may only be a crack in the mental health system. The combination of all of them has created a serious fissure in the system's very foundation.

The stories of my son's life and of my experiences in a mental institution coupled with the evidence from experts in the field should leave no doubt. Add to all that the words of Dr. Lloyd I. Sederer of the New York State Office of Mental Health who refers to the system as "flawed" and calls for legislative action to "repair a broken system and deliver opportunities for healing and recovery for millions of people in this country."[180]

Dr. Sederer's words cry out for people to learn how broken the current mental health system is and do something about it.

Do not sit back and say, "It doesn't affect me." The personal, social and economic costs to all of us are enormous. More than 50 percent of all mental health expenditures are shouldered by the public, and people with serious mental illness are the single largest group receiving Supplemental Security Income.

According to the *Journal of Clinical Psychiatry,* the costs associated with clinical depression alone were $210 billion in 2015 as a result of absenteeism from work, lost productivity and direct treatment costs.[181]

Furthermore, when untreated, mental health issues lead to an increased risk of substance abuse, which creates a significant burden to society.

As an article in *Journal of Food and Drug Analysis* puts it, substance use disorders "contribute to housing instability, homelessness, criminal behaviors (victim or perpetrator) and incarceration, the transmission of HIV due to IV drug use or high-risk sexual behaviors, and unemployment or dependence on welfare. The costs associated with these social problems are staggering, creating an economic burden for governments or payors who spend considerable sums of money on treatments for addiction, medical or psychiatric disorders, and other related problems such as those associated with welfare dependence, unemployment, or involvement in the criminal justice or social service systems."[182]

And, if these social and economic effects are too difficult to visualize, just remember one mother and one son.

Remember my son for whom "healing and recovery" is a vanished dream.

Alan Ross Jacobs was two weeks shy of his 29th birthday when he died—killed by pills.

Allowed to die by mental health professionals that were either incompetent, overworked or undereducated.

Allowed to die by a mother who didn't have enough information to save him, who naively put her faith in the mental health system.

Some who read this will, no doubt, judge me, believing I could have and should have been more proactive. You will never blame me more than I blame myself. That is a pain I live with every day.

I could rationalize, explain why I didn't do things I could have done, but this book is partly an attempt to reduce my guilt and to share what I've kept hidden.

I very rarely tell anyone about my experiences. I don't even tell most people that my son died. Perhaps I don't want that tragedy to define me. Perhaps I don't want the loss of Alan to become a kind of currency to be traded for special treatment. Maybe I don't want to be subjected to the heartfelt comments that often annoy me.

Well-intentioned people will tell me how they dealt with the loss of a husband or wife. It's simply not the same kind of loss. Others will say, "Time heals."

Don't tell me I'll heal. I won't. What I'll do is cope.

At some point, those of us who have lost a child tell ourselves we have to accept the reality, the "new normal." And then we put one foot in front of the other. We do what we have to do.

We even eventually enjoy things, although singing along with a favorite song or laughing at something can still make me feel guilty that I'm alive and Alan isn't. It can still bring me to tears. My tears are triggered by many things.

Shopping for food reduced me to tears for almost a year and still sometimes does. Several years after Alan's death, I still can't eat his favorite foods. It took more than a year before I could look at a picture of Alan, the man, without breaking down. Every time I see a woman holding her brand new baby, the tears flow. Every TV or radio ad for drug rehabilitation hurts like hell.

But, I walk through the sadness.

The mindfulness and deep-breathing techniques I learned in the outpatient program help me get through the worst moments — moments when the pain is so visceral that it doesn't seem possible to keep going. In those moments, I hear Evie's voice saying, "You are the strongest woman I know," and I let myself believe it.

I miss Alan every single day. Sometimes I see him standing in the living room doorway as he so often did. Sometimes lying in bed at night, I feel him holding my hand again. Many times I turn to tell him about something I've seen or heard — a scientific discovery, political stupidity, children's antics. Sometimes I post those things on his Facebook page as if I am having a conversation with him. It's all hard.

The worst is when the truth that he is dead knifes my consciousness. It's sudden and overpowering. I hear an awful sound escape from me as the truth hits: Alan is dead, buried. The life he could have, should have lived is no more.

At those moments when denying the truth is not possible, it once again seems I can't go on. Then I remember I've gotten this far. I've lived these years without him. I haven't got much further to go. And the moment passes.

At other times, the grief makes me feel like a partially inflated balloon that has no string to tether it. At those times, there seems to be nothing that connects me to this world. Like a balloon, I lie still until a breath of air whispers beneath me that there are things that need to be done, responsibilities that need to be fulfilled. The moving air lifts me ever so slightly and rolls me forward.

One of those responsibilities has been writing this book. I needed to keep Alan's memory alive. I needed to do anything I could to prevent others from walking the paths Alan and I walked.

I needed you to know there are things parents can do.

First and foremost, protect your children without suffocating them or making them fearful. When confronted by medical or mental health professionals, remember that you may very well know your children better than they do. Use what you know even if that means bludgeoning the professionals with that knowledge.

Do your homework: research every professional, every pill, every treatment no matter how arduous a task that is. Perhaps the resources at the end of his book can help you do that.

Think of the hundreds upon hundreds of lives that are broken by the mental health system as it is today. Advocate to change that.

Talk to people, write to government officials, volunteer so that victims of addiction and mental illness receive the very best care.

Remember to always listen to those in pain: be a shoulder to lean on without judging.

Remember Alan Ross Jacobs and the life that was robbed from him. Do not let that memory vanish when you close this book. Use the knowledge you have gained to help yourself, your family and others successfully navigate the quicksand of the mental health system.

A "person with mental illness can recover even though the illness is not 'cured'…. [Recovery] is a way of living a satisfying, hopeful, and contributing life even with the limitations caused by illness."[184]

There is always hope.

APPENDIX

The resources below are by no means an exhaustive list of all of the resources that are available. If you take anything away from this section, take this:

There is *always* help available.

Suicide Hotlines

If you fear — or believe — that suicide is your only option, there are people you can talk to 24 hours a day, 365 days a year. Just call one of the phone numbers listed below:

National Suicide Prevention Lifeline
  1-800-273-TALK (8255)
Suicide Prevention Hotline
  1-800-827-7571
Suicide Hotline for the deaf
  1-800-799-4TTY

Crisis Hotlines

In addition to the suicide prevention hotlines listed above, other hotlines are available for a variety of issues:

Dial 211 or visit http://www.211.org/
  Provides a multitude of local support resources and services.
Text SUPPORT to 741-741
  Trained counselors can discuss anything that's on your mind. Free, 24/7, confidential.

1in6

https://1in6.org/helpline

Provides educational information and resources for men who've been sexually abused or assaulted. Chat with a trained advocate through the national helpline for men, available 24/7. Join a weekly chat-based online support group, facilitated by a counselor. 1in6 also serves loved ones and service providers.

National Child Abuse Hotline

1-800-422-4453 Call or text

A centralized call center provides the caller with the option of talking with or texting a counselor. Callers are also connected to a language line that can provide service in over 140 languages.

National Domestic Violence Hotline

1-800-799-7233

Provides 24/7 crisis intervention, safety planning and information on domestic violence.

Drug Abuse National Helpline

1-800-662-4357

Gay and Lesbian National Hotline

1-888-843-4564

Helpline for Gays

1-800-398-GAYS

GriefShare

1-800-395-5755

National Sexual Assault Hotline

1-800-656-HOPE (4673)

National Street Harassment Hotline

1-855-897-5910

Created by Stop Street Harassment, Defend Yourself, and operated by RAINN (Rape, Abuse & Incest National Network), the National Street Harassment Hotline is a resource for those affected by gender-based street harassment. Support is available in English and Spanish.

Teen Hope Line
    1-800-394-HOPE
United Way Crisis Helpline
    1-800-233-HELP

Counseling Services

Families Anonymous
    1-800-736-9805
    This is a twelve-step program for relatives and friends of addicts.
Open Path Psychotherapy Collective
    https://openpathcollective.org/
    Patients pay a one-time fee of $49, and then have lifetime access to
    therapists who charge only $30-60 per session
National Association of Free and Charitable Clinics
    https://www.nafcclinics.org/
Substance Abuse and Mental Health Services Administration Helpline
    1-800-662-HELP (4357)
    TTY: 1-800-487-4889
    This confidential, free, 24-hour-a-day, 365-day-a-year, information
    service, in English and Spanish, for individuals and family members
    facing mental and/or substance use disorders. This service provides
    referrals to local treatment facilities, support groups, and
    community-based organizations. Callers can also order free
    publications and other information. If you have no insurance or are
    underinsured, you will be referred to your state office, which is
    responsible for state-funded treatment programs. In addition, you
    may be referred to facilities that charge on a sliding fee scale or
    accept Medicare or Medicaid.
Find a Health Center, U.S. Department of Health and Human Services
    https://findahealthcenter.hrsa.gov/
    Provides information on federally funded health centers where
    patients pay only what they can afford.
Psychology Today

https://www.psychologytoday.com/us
Psychology Today offers a national directory of therapists, psychiatrists, therapy groups and treatment facility options.
The Association of Psychology Training Clinics
https://www.aptc.org/?module=Members&event=Clinics
Lists clinical training centers that may offer low-cost or free counseling services.
National Alliance on Mental Health (NAMI)
https://www.nami.org/Find-Your-Local-NAMI
Offers free support and education services

Support Groups

Male Survivor https://malesurvivor.org/survivors/
Provides resources and support to male survivors of all forms of sexual abuse, including Weekends of Recovery and peer moderated discussion forums
Mad in America (MIA) Online Parent Support Groups
https://www.madinamerica.com/mia-online-parents-support-group/
NAMI Support Groups
https://www.nami.org/Find-Support/NAMI-Programs

Resources for Mental Health Conditions

National Alliance on Mental Illness (NAMI) Helpline
800-950-NAMI
or text "NAMI" to 741741
Children and Adults with Attention-Deficit/Hyperactivity Disorder (CHADD)
800-233-4050
Provides information and referrals on ADHD, including local support groups.
Anxiety and Depression Association of America (ADAA)
240-485-1001
Provides information on prevention, treatment and symptoms of anxiety, depression and related conditions.

The American Foundation for Suicide Prevention
> 1-888-333-2377
> Provides referrals to support groups, mental health professionals, resources on loss and suicide prevention information.

Treatment and Research Advancements for Borderline Personality Disorder (TARA)
> 1-888-482-7227
> Offers a referral center for information, support, education and treatment options for BPD.

Depression and Bipolar Support Alliance (DBSA)
> 1-800-826-3632
> Provides information on bipolar disorder and depression, offers in-person and online support groups and forums.

International OCD Foundation
> 617-973-5801
> Provides information on OCD and treatment referrals.

Schizophrenia and Related Disorders Alliance of America (SARDAA)
> 240-423-9432
> Maintains the Schizophrenia Anonymous programs, which are self-help groups and are now available as toll free teleconferences.

Sidran Institute
> https://www.sidran.org
> 410-825-8888
> Sidran Institute helps people understand, manage and treat trauma and dissociation and maintains a helpline for information and referrals.

Mental Health Advocacy

Mental Health America (MHA)
> https://www.mentalhealthamerica.net
> For more than 100 years, has been addressing the needs of those living with mental illness and promoting the overall mental health of all Americans.

National Alliance on Mental Illness (NAMI)

> https://www.nami.org
>
> One of the oldest mental health advocacy groups in the United States, NAMI provides mental health support to millions, and leads important awareness campaigns and advocacy and lobbying efforts to help promote mental well-being across the nation.

Active Minds

> https://www.activeminds.org
>
> Supports mental health awareness and education for students. Through education, research, advocacy, and a focus on students and young adults ages 14–25, Active Minds is opening up the conversation about mental health and creating lasting change in the way mental health is talked about, cared for, and valued in the United States.

Project Semicolon

> https://projectsemicolon.com/
>
> Dedicated to the prevention of suicide, Project Suicide raises public awareness, educates communities, and equips people with the right tools to save lives.

Legal Assistance

Legal Services Corporation
> https://www.lsc.gov/
> Legal Services Corporation (LSC) is an independent nonprofit established by Congress to provide financial support for civil legal aid to low-income Americans. LSC promotes equal access to justice by providing funding to 133 independent non-profit legal aid programs in every state, the District of Columbia, and U.S. Territories.

National Disability Rights Network (State Protection and Advocacy Agencies)
> https://www.ndrn.org/
> Protects the civil rights of individuals with disabilities, particularly in hospitals and state prison systems.

Financial Assistance

Allsup, LLC
> https://allsup.com
> 800-279-4357
> Provides non-attorney representation when applying for Social Security Disability Insurance benefits (SSDI).

HealthCare.gov
> https://www.healthcare.gov/
> 1-800-318-2596
> Provides specific information about coverage options in your state, includes private options, high risk pools and other public programs.

Need Help Paying Bills
> https://www.needhelppayingbills.com
> This organization provides information on thousands of financial assistance programs that offer help with everything from medication bill assistance or free healthcare to mortgage debt help to free groceries. Includes information on state and local assistance programs and charity organizations.

NeedyMeds
> http://www.needymeds.org/
> 1-800-503-6897
> The mission of this 5013 non-profit is to help people who cannot afford medicine or healthcare costs. The information at NeedyMeds is available anonymously and free of charge.

Medicine Assistance Tool
> https://medicineassistancetool.org/
> PhRMA's medical assistance tool (MAT) is a search engine tool designed to help patients, caregivers and healthcare providers learn about the resources available through various biopharmaceutical industry programs. Assistance Tool (MAT) is a search engine designed to help patients, caregivers and health care providers learn more about the resources available through the various biopharmaceutical industry programs. MAT is not its own patient assistance program, but rather a search engine for many of the patient assistance resources that the biopharmaceutical industry offers.

Partnership for Prescription Assistance (PPA)
> https://www.pparx.org/
> This free and confidential service helps connect uninsured and underinsured patients who struggle with affordable access to medicines to prescription assistance programs that offer medicines for free or nearly free.

Recommended Reading

"What to do in a Crisis" A NAMI publication
> https://www.nami.org/Find-Support/Living-with-a-Mental-Health-Condition/What-to-Do-In-a-Crisis

Facing Addiction in America: The Surgeon General's Spotlight on Opioids
> https://addiction.surgeongeneral.gov/

The Family Guide to Mental Health Care
> by Lloyd Sederer. W.W. Norton & Company

"To improve mental health treatments, scientists try to dissect the pieces that make them work."

https://www.statnews.com/2019/02/01/back-translation-mental-health-treatments/

"As Suicides Rise, Insurers Find Ways to Deny Mental Health Coverage"

https://www.bloomberg.com/news/features/2019-05-16/insurance-covers-mental-health-but-good-luck-using-it

When Your Adult Child Breaks Your Heart: Coping With Mental Illness, Substance Abuse, And The Problems That Tear Families Apart

by Joel Young, M.D. and Christine Adamac. Lyons Press, 2015.

Unhinged: The Trouble with Psychiatry—A Doctor's Revelations about a Profession in Crisis

by Daniel Carlat, M.D. Free Press, 2010.

Drug Dealer, MD: How Doctors Were Duped, Patients Got Hooked, and Why It's So Hard to Stop

by Anna Lembke, MD. Johns Hopkins University Press, 2016.

Anatomy of an Epidemic: Magic Bullets, Psychiatric Drugs, and the Astonishing Rise of Mental Illness in America

by Robert Whitaker, MD, Crown, 2010.

Mad in America: Bad Science, Bad Medicine, and the Enduring Mistreatment of the Mentally Ill

by Robert Whitaker. Basic Books, 2002.

Mad in America: Science, Psychiatry and Social Justice.

newsletter@madinamerica.com

A weekly online newsletter published by Mad in America, a 501(c)(3) non-profit whose mission is to produce a platform for rethinking psychiatric care.

Substance Abuse Resources

Opioid Overdose Prevention Toolkit

https://store.samhsa.gov/product/Opioid-Overdose-Prevention-Toolkit/SMA18-4742

American Association for the Treatment of Opioid Dependence
http://www.aatod.org/
Narcotics Anonymous
https://www.na.org/
Partnership for Drug-Free Kids Parents Helpline
855-378-4373
Text a Message to 55753
U.S. National Library of Medicine's listing of addiction resources
https://ghr.nlm.nih.gov/condition/opioid-addiction#resources

REFERENCES

Note: The following references were cited at various places in the text of the book. Some references are direct links to websites. In some cases, because mental health research and statistics are constantly changing, the figures presented in the book at the time of its writing are no longer reflected on the cited pages. The references below indicate when the website was originally cited or what the web page presented as the original publication date. Efforts were made to link directly to original sources or studies whenever possible.

1. Metzl, Jonathan M. , MD, PhD, and Kenneth T. MacLeish, PhD. "Mental Illness, Mass Shootings, and the Politics of American Firearms." *American Journal of Public Health,* vol. 105, no. 2, Feb. 2015, pp. 240-249. https://www.ncbi.nlm.nih.gov/pmc/articles/PMC4318286/.
2. Mental Health. gov. "Mental Health Myths and Facts." Last updated Aug. 29, 2017 https://www.mentalhealth.gov/basics/mental-health-myths-facts.
3. Krans, Brian. "Stigma Still a Major Hurdle in Getting People the Mental Health Care They Need." Healthline. March 2, 2014. https://www.healthline.com/health-news/mental-health-treatment-hindered-by-stigma-030214#1

4. World Health Organization. "Mental Disorders affect one in four people." Oct. 2001, http://www.who.int/whr/2001/media_centre/press_release/en/
5. Fisher, Daniel M.D. Ph.D. "People Can Recover from Mental Illness." https://power2u.org/people-can-recover-from-mental-illness/
6. World Health Organization. "Mental Disorders affect one in four people." Oct. 2001, http://www.who.int/whr/2001/media_centre/press_release/en/
7. U.S. Department of Health and Human Services, Office of Adolescent Health Care. "Access to Adolescent Mental Health Care." https://www.hhs.gov/ash/oah/adolescent-development/mental-health/access-to-mental-health-care/index.html
8. National Institute of Mental Health. "Mental Health Information." Updated Feb. 2019, https://www.nimh.nih.gov/health/statistics/mental-illness.shtml
9. Becker's Hospital Review. "Amid shortage, number of psychiatric beds in US down 13% from 2010." https://www.beckershospitalreview.com/patient-flow/amid-shortage-number-of-psychiatric-beds-in-us-down-13-from-2010.html
10. Merritt Hawkins. "The Silent Shortage A White Paper Examining Supply, Demand and Recruitment Trends in Psychiatry" https://www.merritthawkins.com/uploadedFiles/merritthawkins_whitepaper_psychiatry_2018.pdf
11. National Institute of Mental Health. "U.S. Leading Categories of Diseases/Disorders." https://www.nimh.nih.gov/health/statistics/disability/us-leading-categories-of-diseases-disorders.shtml
12. Bacon, John. "'We are losing too many Americans': Suicides, drug overdoses rise as US life expectancy drops." https://www.usatoday.com/story/news/2018/11/29/us-life-expectancy-suicide-50-year-peak-and-drugs-cause-death/2146829002/

13. Curtin, Sally C., M.A., Margaret Warner, Ph.D., and Holly Hedegaard, M.D., M.S.P.H."Increase in Suicide in the United States, 1999–2014." NCHS Data Brief No. 241. April 2016. https://www.cdc.gov/nchs/products/databriefs/db241.htm

14. National Institute of Mental Health. "U.S. Leading Categories of Diseases/Disorders." https://www.nimh.nih.gov/health/statistics/disability/us-leading-categories-of-diseases-disorders.shtml

15. Anxiety and Depression Association of America. "Facts and Statistics." https://adaa.org/about-adaa/press-room/facts-statistics

16. Winston, Robert and Rebecca Chicot. "The importance of early bonding on the long-term mental health and resilience of children." *London Journal of Primary Care* *https://www.ncbi.nlm.nih.gov/pmc/articles/PMC5330336/*

17. Laldin, Myra. "The Psychology of Belonging (and Why It Matters). https://www.learningandthebrain.com/blog/psychology-of-belonging/

18. Hesdhmat, Shahram Ph.D. "What is Confirmation Bias?" *Psychology Today* April 23, 2015 https://www.psychologytoday.com/us/blog/science-choice/201504/what-is-confirmation-bias

19. Tull, Matthew, Ph.D. "Recognizing Hyperarousal Symptoms in PTSD." VeryWellMind. https://www.verywellmind.com/hyperarousal-2797362

20. Centers for Disease Control. "Data and Statistics About ADHD." https://www.cdc.gov/ncbddd/adhd/data.html

21. Centers for Disease Control. "Data and Statistics About ADHD." https://www.cdc.gov/ncbddd/adhd/data.html

22. CBS News. "Doctors sound the alarm on 'opioid alternative' gabapentin." April 2, 2018, https://www.cbsnews.com/news/gabapentin-opioid-alternative-doctors-warning-about-drug/

23. Alexander, Caroline. "Word War I: 100 Years Later." *Smithsonian Magazine, September 2010,* https://www.smithsonianmag.com/history/the-shock-of-war-55376701/

24. Jones, Joshua A. "A brief history of PTSD: The evolution of our understanding." *Military 1,* September 3, 2013 https://www.military1.com/army/article/405058-a-brief-history-of-ptsd-the-evolution-of-our-understanding/

25. Crocq, Marc-Antoine, M.D. "From shell shock and war neurosis to posttraumatic stress disorder: a history of psychotraumatology." *Dialogues in Clinical Neuroscience,* vol. 2, no. 1, March 2000, pp. 47-54 https://www.ncbi.nlm.nih.gov/pmc/articles/PMC3181586/

26. Friedman, Matthew J., M.D., Ph.D. "PTSD History and Overview." U.S. Department of Veterans Affairs. PTSD: National Center for PTSD. https://www.ptsd.va.gov/professional/treat/essentials/history_ptsd.asp

27. National Institute of Mental Health. "Post-Traumatic Stress Disorder." https://www.nimh.nih.gov/health/topics/post-traumatic-stress-disorder-ptsd/index.shtml

28. Holt, Billie Lynn. "June is PTSD Awareness Month." *NTI@Home: Advocacy, Awareness and Job Information for Americans with Disabilities and Disabled Veterans,* http://blog.nticentral.org/2017/06/june-is-ptsd-awareness-month.html

29. Centers for Disease Control, "Data and Statistics About ADHD" https://www.cdc.gov/ncbddd/adhd/data.html

30. Thomas, Liji, M.D. "One in 13 children affected by PTSD, according to landmark study." *News Medical Life Sciences* https://www.news-medical.net/news/20190222/One-in-13-children-affected-by-PTSD-according-to-landmark-study.aspx

31. Dworkin, Emily R., Suvarna Menon, Jonathan Bystrynski and Nicole Allen. "Sexual assault victimization and psychopathology: A review and meta-analysis." *Clinical Psychology Review,* vol. 56, June 2017, pp. 65-81
https://www.sciencedirect.com/science/article/pii/S027273581730008 80

32. Hurd, Ryan. "What Are the Psychological Causes of Bedwetting?" Livestrong.com
https://www.livestrong.com/article/97067-psychological-causes-bedwetting/

33. National Institute of Mental Health. "What is post-traumatic stress disorder, or PTSD?"
https://www.nimh.nih.gov/health/publications/post-traumatic-stress-disorder-ptsd/index.shtml

34. King, Sandra. "New York State Mental Health Involuntary Commitment Laws." https://legalbeagle.com/6759290-new-health-involuntary-commitment-laws.html

35. Heshmat, Shahram, Ph.D. "What Is Confirmation Bias?" *Psychology Today,* April 23, 2015
https://www.psychologytoday.com/us/blog/science-choice/201504/what-is-confirmation-bias

36. Folk, James, and Marilyn Folk, BScN "One In Four Older Adults Prescribed Risky Long-term Benzodiazepine Medication"
https://www.anxietycentre.com/anxiety/research/older-adults-prescribed-risky-long-term-benzodiazepine-medication.shtml

37. New York State Office of Mental Health. "Rights of Inpatients in New York State Office of Mental Health Psychiatric Centers."
https://www.omh.ny.gov/omhweb/patientrights/inpatient_rts.htm

38. *Natural News.* "Aspartame's neurological side effects include blurred vision, headaches, seizures and more."
https://www.naturalnews.com/035242_aspartame_side_effects_neurological.html

39. clinical-depression.co.uk. "Depression and Your Sense of Control." https://www.clinical-depression.co.uk/dlp/understanding-depression/depression-and-your-sense-of-control/

40. New York State Office of Mental Health. "Rights of Inpatients in New York State Office of Mental Health Psychiatric Centers." https://www.omh.ny.gov/omhweb/patientrights/inpatient_rts.htm

41. New York State Office of Mental Health. "Rights of Inpatients in New York State Office of Mental Health Psychiatric Centers." https://www.omh.ny.gov/omhweb/patientrights/inpatient_rts.htm

42. New York State Office of Mental Health. "Rights of Inpatients in New York State Office of Mental Health Psychiatric Centers" https://www.omh.ny.gov/omhweb/patientrights/inpatient_rts.htm

43. Carroll , Robert, Chris Metcalfe and David Gunnell. "Hospital Presenting Self-Harm and Risk of Fatal and Non-Fatal Repetition: Systematic Review and Meta-Analysis" Chris Metcalfe, David Gunnell PLOS One February 28, 2014 https://www.ncbi.nlm.nih.gov/pmc/articles/PMC3938547/

44. Bostwick, J. Michael M.D., Chaitanya Pabbati, M.D., Jennifer R. Geske, M.S., Alastair J. McKean, M.D."Suicide Attempt as a Risk Factor for Completed Suicide: Even More Lethal Than We Knew." https://ajp.psychiatryonline.org/doi/full/10.1176/appi.ajp.2016.1507 0854

45. Vaiva, Guillaume et al. "ALGOS: the development of a randomized controlled trial testing a case management algorithm designed to reduce suicide risk among suicide attempters." *BMC psychiatry* vol. 11 1. 2 Jan. 2011 https://www.ncbi.nlm.nih.gov/pmc/articles/PMC3023738/

46. Oquendo, Maria and Enrique Baca-Garcia. "Suicidal behavior disorder as a diagnostic entity in the DSM-5 classification system: advantages outweigh limitations." *World Psychiatry* 2014 Jun. https://www.ncbi.nlm.nih.gov/pmc/articles/PMC4102277/

47. Morrill, Zenobia. "Meta-Analysis Finds Asking About Suicidal Thoughts Does Not Predict Suicide." *MAD In America: Science,*

Psychiatry and Social Justice February 11, 2019
https://www.madinamerica.com/2019/02/meta-analysis-finds-asking-suicidal-thoughts-not-predict-suicide/

48. McHugh, C. M., A. Corderoy, C.J. Ryan, I.B. Hickie, &M.M. Large. "Association between suicidal ideation and suicide: meta-analyses of odds ratios, sensitivity, specificity and positive predictive valueI *BJPsych* open
https://www.ncbi.nlm.nih.gov/pmc/articles/PMC6401538/

49. Oquendo, Maria and Enrique Baca-Garcia. "Suicidal behavior disorder as a diagnostic entity in the DSM-5 classification system: advantages outweigh limitations." *World Psychiatry.* 2014 Jun; 13(2): 128–130.
https://www.ncbi.nlm.nih.gov/pmc/articles/PMC4102277/

50. Sharma, T, L.S. Guski, N. Freund, P.C. Gotzsche "Suicidality and aggression during antidepressant treatment: systematic review and meta-analyses based on clinical study reports." *BMJ.* Jan 27, 2016.
https://www.bmj.com/content/352/bmj.i65

51. Gibbons, Robert D., PhD, Dr. C. Hendricks Brown, PhD, Dr. Kwan Hur, Phd, Dr. John M. Davis, MD, and Dr. J. John Mann, MD. *Arch Gen Psychiatry.* 2012 Jun. "Suicidal Thoughts and Behavior With Antidepressant Treatment Reanalysis of the Randomized Placebo-Controlled Studies of Fluoxetine and Venlafaxine."
https://jamanetwork.com/journals/jamapsychiatry/fullarticle/1151018

52. Jacobson, Roni. "Many Antidepressant Studies Found Tainted by Pharma Company Influence." *Scientific American.*
https://www.scientificamerican.com/article/many-antidepressant-studies-found-tainted-by-pharma-company-influence/?redirect=1

53. Hengartner, Michael P. and Martin Plöderl. "Newer-Generation Antidepressants and Suicide Risk in Randomized Controlled Trials: A Re-Analysis of the FDA Database." *Psychotherapy and Psychosomatics.* March 15, 2019
https://www.karger.com/Article/FullText/501215

54. Kirsch, Irving. "Antidepressants and the Placebo Effect." *Z Psychol.* 2014. https://www.ncbi.nlm.nih.gov/pmc/articles/PMC4172306/

55. U.S. National Library of Medicine. "ASSIP, Attempted Suicide Short Intervention Program. Two Year Follow-Up Study (ASSIP)" https://clinicaltrials.gov/ct2/show/study/NCT02505373

56. Hickey, Phil, Ph.D. "Involuntary Mental Health Commitments." *Behaviorism and Mental Health.* March 20, 2014 http://behaviorismandmentalhealth.com/2014/03/20/involuntary-mental-health-commitments/

57. Hickey, Phil, Ph.D. "Involuntary Mental Health Commitments." Behaviorism and Mental Health. March 20, 2014 http://behaviorismandmentalhealth.com/2014/03/20/involuntary-mental-health-commitments/

58. U.S. National Library of Medicine. "ASSIP, Attempted Suicide Short Intervention Program. Two Year Follow-Up Study (ASSIP)." https://clinicaltrials.gov/ct2/show/NCT02505373

59. U.S. National Library of Medicine. "ASSIP, Attempted Suicide Short Intervention Program. Two Year Follow-Up Study (ASSIP)." https://clinicaltrials.gov/ct2/show/NCT02505373

60. Ghahramanlou-Holloway, Marjan, PhD and Laura L. Neely, PsyD. "A cognitive-behavioral strategy for preventing suicide" *Current Psychiatry.* 2014 August. https://www.mdedge.com/psychiatry/article/85951/depression/cognitive-behavioral-strategy-preventing-suicide

61. Behavioral Research and Therapy Clinics University of Washington. "Dialectical Behavioral Therapy." http://depts.washington.edu/uwbrtc/about-us/dialectical-behavior-therapy/

62. Deci, E. L., & Ryan, R. M. "Facilitating optimal motivation and psychological well-being across life's domains." *Canadian Psychology/Psychologie Canadienne.* 2008. https://selfdeterminationtheory.org/SDT/documents/2008_DeciRyan_CanPsy_Eng.pdf

63. Deci, E. L., & Ryan, R. M. "Facilitating optimal motivation and psychological well-being across life's domains." *Canadian Psychology/Psychologie Canadienne.* 2008. https://selfdeterminationtheory.org/SDT/documents/2008_DeciRyan_CanPsy_Eng.pdf

64. Suicide Prevention Resource Center. "Suicide Attempts and Dying by Suicide." March 10, 2017. http://www.sprc.org/news/suicide-attempts-dying-suicide

65. Brody, Jane. "After a Suicide Attempt, the Risk of Another Try." *The New York Times.* Nov. 7, 2016 https://www.nytimes.com/2016/11/08/well/live/after-a-suicide-attempt-the-risk-of-another-try.html

66. NIATx. "Use the Spirit of Motivational Interviewing during the First Contact." http://www.niatx.net/toolkits/provider/PP_UseMIFirstContact.pdf

67. Dixon, Lisa B., Yael Holoshitz and Ilana Nossel. "Treatment engagement of individuals experiencing mental illness: review and update." *World Psychiatry.* February 2016. https://www.ncbi.nlm.nih.gov/pmc/articles/PMC4780300/

68. Suicide Prevention Resource Center. "Suicide Attempts and Dying by Suicide." March 10, 2017. http://www.sprc.org/news/suicide-attempts-dying-suicide

69. Valva, Guillaume, Michel Walter, Abeer S Al Arab, Philippe Courtet, Frank Bellivier, Anne Laure Demarty, Stephane Duhem, Francois Ducrocq, Patrick Goldstein and Christian Libersa. "ALGOS:the development of a randomized controlled trial testing a case management algorithm designed to reduce suicide risk among suicide attempters." *BMC Psychiatry.* 2011. https://bmcpsychiatry.biomedcentral.com/articles/10.1186/1471-244X-11-1

70. Kamal, Rabah. "What are the current costs and outcomes related to mental health and substance abuse disorders?" Peterson-Kaiser Health System Tracker. July 31, 2017

https://www.healthsystemtracker.org/chart-collection/current-costs-outcomes-related-mental-health-substance-abuse-disorders/

71. Corrigan, Patrick W., G. Druss, Deborah A. Perlick ."The Impact of Mental Illness Stigma on Seeking and Participating in Mental Health Care." *Psychological Science in the Public Interest.* Sept. 3, 2014 http://journals.sagepub.com/stoken/rbtfl/dDpyhM2zRi.Fg/full

72. Mojtabai, Ramin, MD, PHD, MPH, Mark Olfson, MD, MPH, Nancy A. Sampson, BA, Robert Jin, MA, Benjamin Druss, MD, MPH, Philip S. Want, MD. Dr. PH, Keneth B. Wells, MD, MPH, Harold A. Pincus, MD, and Ronald C. Kessler, PhD "Barriers to Mental Health Treatment: Results from the National Comorbidity Survey Replication (NCS-R)." *Psychol Med.* 2011 August www.ncbi.nlm.nih.gov/pmc/articles/PMC3128692/

73. Mukherjee, Sy. "Study: Americans Just Can't Afford Mental Health Treatment"" Sy Mukherjee. Jan 24, 2013. Think Progress https://thinkprogress.org/study-americans-just-cant-afford-mental-health-treatment-bf0a3c3d5b2d/

74. Hooper, Deona, MSW. "Top Five Barriers to Mental Health Treatment." May 2, 2017 SWHELPER. https://www.socialworkhelper.com/2017/05/02/top-five-barriers-mental-health-treatment/

75. Rauch, Joseph. "How Much Does Therapy Cost? (And Why Is It So Expensive?)" Talkspace. https://www.talkspace.com/blog/how-much-does-therapy-cost-and-why-is-it-crazy-expensive/

76. Raphelson, Samantha. "How the Loss of U.S. Psychiatric Hospitals Led to a Mental Health Crisis." Nov 30, 2017. Health News Florida. https://health.wusf.usf.edu/post/how-loss-us-psychiatric-hospitals-led-mental-health-crisis#stream/0

77. B., Minaa. "Mental Health Treatment Is A Privilege Many People Can't Afford." *Huffington Post.* 07/28/2015 Updated Jul 28, 2016 https://www.huffpost.com/entry/mental-health-treatment-is-a-privilege-many-people-cant-afford_b_7805248

78. Piper, Kip. "Hospitalizations for Mental Health and Substance Abuse Disorders: Costs, Length of Stay, Patient Mix, and Payor Mix." June 25, 2011. Piper Report. https://piperreport.com/blog/2011/06/25/hospitalizations-for-mental-health-and-substance-abuse-disorders-costs-length-of-stay-patient-mix-and-payor-mix/

79. Szabo, Liz. "Cost of not caring: Nowhere to go. " *USA Today.* January 12, 2015 https://www.usatoday.com/story/news/nation/2014/05/12/mental-health-system-crisis/7746535/

80. Raphelson, Samantha. "How the Loss of Psychiatric Hospitals Led To A Mental Health Crisis." November 30, 2017. NPR. https://www.npr.org/2017/11/30/567477160/how-the-loss-of-u-s-psychiatric-hospitals-led-to-a-mental-health-crisis

81. "Amid shortage of psychiatric beds, mentally ill face long waits for treatment." August 2, 2106. PBS News Hour https://www.pbs.org/newshour/nation/amid-shortage-psychiatric-beds-mentally-ill-face-long-waits-treatment

82. Torrey, E. Fuller, M.D. "A Dearth of Psychiatric Beds." *Psychiatric Times.* February 25 2016 http://www.psychiatrictimes.com/psychiatric-emergencies/dearth-psychiatric-beds

83. Burton, Evelyn. "Md.'s psychiatric bed shortage detrimental to patients and community." *The Baltimore Sun.* April 24, 2018. https://www.baltimoresun.com/opinion/op-ed/bs-ed-op-0425-bed-shortage-20180424-story.html

84. Hanrahan, Laura M.D. "The Revolving Door: A Look at Factors Effecting Readmission to Inpatient Psychiatry." University of Buffalo https://ubmm.med.buffalo.edu/uploads/MMU3/01292016%20The%20Revolving%20Door.pdf

85. Heslin, Kevin C. Ph.D. and Audrey J. Weiss, Ph.D. "Hospital Readmissions Involving Psychiatric Disorders, 2012."

https://www.hcup-us.ahrq.gov/reports/statbriefs/sb189-Hospital-Readmissions-Psychiatric-Disorders-2012.pdf

86. Institute of Medicine (US) Committee on Crossing the Quality Chasm: Adaptation to Mental Health and Addictive Disorders. Improving the Quality of Health Care for Mental and Substance-Use Conditions: Quality Chasm Series. Washington, D.C.: National Academies Press, 2006.
https://www.ncbi.nlm.nih.gov/books/NBK19817/

87. Finnerty, Molly MD"The Quality Concern: Behavioral Health Inpatient Readmissions." Bureau of Evidence Based Services and Implementation Science New York State Office of Mental Health. June 21, 2012.
https://www.omh.ny.gov/omhweb/psyckes_medicaid/initiatives/hospital/learning_collaborative_2013/Quality_Concern.pdf

88. "Enhancing Mental Health Care Transitions Reduces Unnecessary Costly Readmissions." Health Catalyst. May 25, 2017
https://www.healthcatalyst.com/success_stories/mental-health-readmission-rates-allina

89. Finnerty, Molly MD"The Quality Concern: Behavioral Health Inpatient Readmissions." Bureau of Evidence Based Services and Implementation Science New York State Office of Mental Health. June 21, 2012.
https://www.omh.ny.gov/omhweb/psyckes_medicaid/initiatives/hospital/learning_collaborative_2013/Quality_Concern.pdf

90. Agency for Healthcare Research and Quality. "Management Strategies to Reduce Psychiatric Readmissions." U.S. Department of Health and Human Services. September 4, 2014
https://effectivehealthcare.ahrq.gov/topics/psychiatric-readmissions/research-protocol/

91. Institute of Medicine (US) Committee on Crossing the Quality Chasm: Adaptation to Mental Health and Addictive Disorders. *Improving the Quality of Health Care for Mental and Substance-Use Conditions: Quality Chasm Series.* Washington, D.c.: National

Academies Press, 2006.
https://www.ncbi.nlm.nih.gov/books/NBK19817/

92. Lindsey, Michael, Wendy Patterson, Kevin Ray, Patrick Roohan "Potentially Preventable Hospital Readmissions among Medicaid Recipients with Mental Health and/or Substance Abuse Health Conditions Compared with All Others: New York State, 2007." New York State Department of Health.
https://www.health.ny.gov/health_care/managed_care/reports/statistics_data/3hospital_readmissions_mentahealth.pdf

93. Shinkman, Ron. "Readmissions lead to $41.3B in additional hospital costs." *Fierce Healthcare.* April 20, 2014
https://www.fiercehealthcare.com/finance/readmissions-lead-to-41-3b-additional-hospital-costs

94. The 2018 *OPEN MINDS* State-By-State Guide To Estimating The Number Of Psychiatrists: An *OPEN MINDS* Market Intelligence Report" May 22, 2018
https://www.openminds.com/store/the-2018-open-minds-state-by-state-guide-to-estimating-the-number-of-psychiatrists-an-open-minds-market-intelligence-report/

95. "New Study Shows 60 Percent of U.S. Counties Without a Single Psychiatrist." New American Economy. October 23, 2017
https://www.newamericaneconomy.org/press-release/new-study-shows-60-percent-of-u-s-counties-without-a-single-psychiatrist/

96. Kamal, Rabah. "What are the current costs and outcomes related to mental health and substance abuse disorders?" Peterson-Kaiser Health System Tracker. July 31, 2017
https://www.healthsystemtracker.org/chart-collection/current-costs-outcomes-related-mental-health-substance-abuse-disorders/

97. "2017 Review of Physician and Advanced Practitioner Recruiting Incentives." Merritt Hawkins.
https://www.merritthawkins.com/uploadedFiles/MerrittHawkins/Pdf/2017_Physician_Incentive_Review_Merritt_Hawkins.pdf

98. "Mental Health Care Health Professional Shortage Areas (HPSAs)." Henry K. Kaiser Family Foundation https://www.kff.org/other/state-indicator/mental-health-care-health-professional-shortage-areas-hpsas/?currentTimeframe=0&sortModel=%7B%22colId%22:%22Location%22,%22sort%22:%22asc%22%7D

99. Sederer, Lloyd. "Where Have All the Psychiatrists Gone?" *U.S. News and World Report*. Sept 15, 2015 https://www.usnews.com/opinion/blogs/policy-dose/2015/09/15/the-us-needs-more-psychiatrists-to-meet-mental-health-demands

100. Kelmenson, Lawrence M.D. "How Psychiatry Evolved Into A Religion." *Mad in America: Science, Psychiatry and Social Justice*. November 27, 2017. https://www.madinamerica.com/2017/11/how-psychiatry-evolved-into-a-religion/

101. Lambert, M.J. "Maximizing Psychotherapy Outcome beyond Evidence-Based Medicine." *Psychotherapy and Psychosomatics*. 2017;86:80-89 https://www.karger.com/Article/FullText/455170#

102. Lambert, Michal J. "Outcomes in psychotherapy: The past and important advances." *Psychotherapy*, 50(1), 42–51 https://pdfs.semanticscholar.org/03c0/6e775fb6ad3eb3a97647befba7 54c2fe708c.pdf

103. Lambert, M.J. "Maximizing Psychotherapy Outcome beyond Evidence-Based Medicine." *Psychotherapy and Psychosomatics*. December 7, 2016 https://www.karger.com/Article/Pdf/455170

104. Whipple, J. L., & Lambert, M. J. "Outcome measures for practice." *Annual Review of Clinical Psychology*. 2011. https://www.researchgate.net/profile/Lambert_Michael/publication/2 62791316_Outcome_assessment_for_clinical_practice/links/54aae2f 30cf2bce6aa1d78f6/Outcome-assessment-for-clinical-practice.pdf

105. Kächele, H. and J. Schachter. "On side effects, destructive processes, and negative outcomes in psychoanalytic therapies: Why is it difficult for psychoanalysts to acknowledge and address treatment failures?" *Contemporary Psychoanalysis*. 2014. https://www.researchgate.net/publication/273795791_On_Side_Effe

cts_Destructive_Processes_and_Negative_Outcomes_in_Psychoanal
ytic_Therapies_Why_Is_It_Difficult_for_Psychoanalysts_to_Ackno
wledge_and_Address_Treatment_Failures

106. Werbart, Andrzej, Camilla von Below, Karin Engqvist & Sofia Lind. "It was like having half of the patient in therapy": Therapists of nonimproved patients looking back on their work, *Psychotherapy Research.* 2018. https://www.tandfonline.com/doi/full/10.1080/10503307.2018.1453621

107. Smith, Brendan L. "Psychologists need more training in suicide risk assessment" American Psychological Association. April 2014 http://www.apa.org/monitor/2014/04/suicide-risk.aspx

108. National Alliance on Mental Illness. "LGBTQ." https://www.nami.org/Find-Support/LGBTQ

109. "Facts about Veteran Suicide" VA Suicide Prevention Program. July 2016. https://www.va.gov/opa/publications/factsheets/Suicide_Prevention_FactSheet_New_VA_Stats_070616_1400.pdf

110. SAMHSA/CSAT Treatment Improvement Protocols Rockville (MD): Substance Abuse and Mental Health Services Administration (US); 1993- https://www.ncbi.nlm.nih.gov/books/NBK82999/

111. SAMHSA/CSAT Treatment Improvement Protocols Rockville (MD): Substance Abuse and Mental Health Services Administration (US); 1993- https://www.ncbi.nlm.nih.gov/books/NBK82999/

112. SAMHSA. "Recovery and Recovery Support." U.S. Department of Health and Human Services. May 17, 2019. https://www.samhsa.gov/find-help/recovery

113. Sutherland, Louis. *Magic Bullets: The Story of Man's Valiant Struggle against Enemy Microbes.* Little, Brown, 1956: Boston.

114. Whitaker, Robert. *Anatomy of an Epidemic: Magic Bullets, Psychiatric Drugs, and the Astonishing Rise of Mental Illness in America.* Crown Publishing, 2010: New York.

115. Horgan, John. "Are Psychiatric Medications Making Us Sicker." *The Chronicle of Higher Education.* September 18, 2011
https://www.chronicle.com/article/Are-Psychiatric-Medications/128976

116. Vittengl J.R. "Poorer Long-Term Outcomes among Persons with Major Depressive Disorder Treated with Medication." *Psychotherapy and Psychosomatics.* September 2017
https://www.karger.com/Article/Abstract/479162

117. Fava G.A. and C. Rafanelli. "Iatrogenic Factors in Psychopathology." *Psychotherapy and Psychomatics.* June 2019
https://www.karger.com/Article/FullText/500151

118. Maslej, M.M., B.M. Bokler, M.J. Russel, K. Eaton, Z. Durisko, S.D. Hollon, G.M. Swanson, J.A. Thomason, B.H. Mulsant and P.W. Andrews. "The Mortality and Myocardial Effects of Antidepressants Are Moderated by Preexisting Cardiovascular Disease: A Meta-Analysis." *Psychotherapy and Psychosomatics.* October 2017
https://www.karger.com/Article/Abstract/477940#

119. Kunutsor, S.K., S. Seidu and K. Khunti. "Depression, antidepressant use, and risk of venous thromboembolism: systematic review and meta-analysis of published observational evidence." *Annals of Medicine.* September 2018.
https://www.ncbi.nlm.nih.gov/pubmed/30001640

120. Kelmenson, Lawrence M.D. "The Three Types of Psychiatric Drugs – A Doctor's Guide for Consumers." *Mad in America.* June 9, 2019.
https://www.madinamerica.com/2019/06/the-three-types-of-psychiatric-drugs-a-doctors-guide-for-consumers/

121. Levin, Madeline, MPH, Nicolas J. Jury, PhD, Kousha Mohseni, MS, and Varuna Srinivasan, MBBS MPH. "Do Antidepressants Increase Suicide Attempts? Do They Have Other Risks?" National Center for

Health Research. http://www.center4research.org/antidepressants-increase-suicide-attempts-risks/

122. Harris, Gardiner. "Psychiatrists Top List in Drug Maker Gifts. " *The New York Times, june 27, 2007* https://www.nytimes.com/2007/06/27/health/psychology/27doctors.html

123. Angell, Marcia. M.D. "Illusions of Psychiatry." *New York Review of Books.* July 14, 2011. https://www.nybooks.com/articles/2011/07/14/illusions-of-psychiatry/

124. Fournier, Jay C., M.A., Robert J. DeRubeis, Ph.S. Steven D. Hollon, Ph.D., *et al.* "Antidepressant Drug effects and Depression Severity: A Patient-Level Meta-Analysis" *JAMA* January 6, 2010 https://www.ncbi.nlm.nih.gov/pmc/articles/PMC3712503/

125. Cowen, Philip J. and Michael Browning. "What has serotonin to do with depression?" *World Psychiatry.* June 2015 https://www.ncbi.nlm.nih.gov/pmc/articles/PMC4471964/

126. Whitaker, Robert. *Anatomy of an Epidemic: Magic Bullets, Psychiatric Drugs, and the Astonishing Rise of Mental Illness in America.* Crown Publishing, 2010: New York.

127. "Depression: How effective are antidepressants?" InformedHealth.org. January 28, 2015 https://www.ncbi.nlm.nih.gov/books/NBK361016/

128. Locher, Cosima PhD, Helen Koechlin, MSc, Sean R. Zion, MA, et al. " Efficacy and Safety of Selective Serotonin Reuptake Inhibitors, Serotonin-Norepinephrine Reuptake Inhibitors, and Placebo for Common Psychiatric Disorders Among Children and Adolescents." October 2017 JAMA Psychiatry https://www.ncbi.nlm.nih.gov/pmc/articles/PMC5667359/

129. Lacasse, Jeffrey R. and Jonathan Leo. "Serotonin and Depression: A Disconnect between the Advertisements and the Scientific Literature." *PLoS Med.* December 2005 https://www.ncbi.nlm.nih.gov/pmc/articles/PMC1277931/

130. Kravitz, R.L., R.M. Epstein, M.D. Feldman, C.E. Franz, R. Azari, M.S. Wilkes, L. Hinton and P.Franks. "Influence of patients' requests for direct-to-consumer advertised antidepressents: a randomized controlled trial." *JAMA*. 2005 Apr 27
https://jamanetwork.com/journals/jama/fullarticle/200780

131. Kam, Katherine. "Can Antidepressants Work for Me?"
https://www.webmd.com/depression/features/are-antidepressants-effective#1

132. Angell, Marcia. M.D. "Illusions of Psychiatry." *New York Review of Books*. July 14, 2011
https://www.nybooks.com/articles/2011/07/14/illusions-of-psychiatry/

133. Oaklander, Mandy. "The Anti Antidepressant." *Time*. July 27,2017.
https://time.com/magazine/us/4876068/august-7th-2017-vol-190-no-6-u-s/

134. Craft, Lynette L. and Frank M. Pena. "The Benefits of Exercise for the Clinically Depressed."
https://pdfs.semanticscholar.org/6a1c/93739c9dfbf58f39afb6827592942b9f9309.pdf?_ga=2.91744410.1804520893.1555621193-1690520476.1555621193

135. Schuch, F.B., D. Vancampfort, J. Richards, S. Rosenbaum, P.B. Ward and B. Stubbs. "Exercise as a treatment for depression: A meta-analysis adjusting for publication bias." J Psychiatr Res. 2016 Jun;77:42-51
https://www.ncbi.nlm.nih.gov/pubmed/26978184

136. Harvey, Samuel B., F.R.A.N.Z.C.P., Ph.D., Simon Overland, Ph.D., Stephani L. Hatch, Ph.D.,Simon Wessely, F.R.C.Psych., M.D., Arnstein Mykletun, Ph.D. and Matthew Hotopf, F.R.C.Psych., Ph.D. "Exercise and the Prevention of Depression: Results of the HUNT Cohort Study." *The American Journal of Psychiatry*. October 2017
https://ajp.psychiatryonline.org/doi/full/10.1176/appi.ajp.2017.16111223?mobileUi=0&

137. Blumenthal, James A. Ph.D., Patrick J. Smith, Ph.D., and Benson M. Hoffman, Ph.D."Is Exercise a Viable Treatment for Depression?" *ACSMs Health Fit Journal.* July/August 2012. https://www.ncbi.nlm.nih.gov/pmc/articles/PMC3674785/

138. Seaman, Andrew M. "Mindfulness therapy works for recurrent depression." Reuters Health https://www.reuters.com/article/us-health-depression-mindfulness-idUSKCN0XQ2L0

139. Soh, Nerissa L. and Garry Walter. "Tryptophan and depression: can diet alone be the answer?" January 5 2011 *Acta Neuropsychiatrica.* https://onlinelibrary.wiley.com/doi/full/10.1111/j.1601-5215.2010.00508.x

140. Coppen, A. and C. Bolander-Gouaille. "Treatment of depression: time to consider folic acid and vitamin B12." *Journal of Psychopharmacology.* January 2005. https://www.researchgate.net/publication/8060947_Treatment_of_depression_Time_to_consider_folic_acid_and_Vitamin_B12

141. Fava, M. and D. Mischoulon. "Folate in depression: efficacy, safety, differences in formulations, and clinical issues." *Alternative Medicine Review.* April 2010. http://go.galegroup.com.arktos.nyit.edu/ps/i.do?p=AONE&u=nysl_li_nyinstc&id=GALE|A2

142. Skarupski, Kimberly A., Christine Tangney, Hong Li, Bichun Ouyang, Denis A, Evans, and Martha Clare Morris. "Longitudinal association of vitamin B-6, folate, and vitamin B-12 with depressive symptoms among older adults over time." *the American Journal of Clinical Nutrition.* June 2, 2010 https://academic.oup.com/ajcn/article/92/2/330/4597287

143. Herzog, Hal Ph.D. "A Strange Relationship Between Vegetarianism and Depression" by Hal Herzog, Ph.D. P*sychology Today.* December 4, 2018 https://www.psychologytoday.com/us/blog/animals-and-us/201812/strange-relationship-between-vegetarianism-and-depression

144. Doctors Health Press Editorial Team. "How Effective Is Omega-3 for Depression?" Doctors Health Press. March 20, 2018. https://www.doctorshealthpress.com/brain-function-articles/omega-3-natural-mood-stabilizer-for-depression/
145. Bergland, Christopher. "The Microbiome-Gut-Brain Axis Relies on Your Vagus Nerve." *Psychology Today.* August 23, 2017. https://www.psychologytoday.com/us/blog/the-athletes-way/201708/the-microbiome-gut-brain-axis-relies-your-vagus-nerve
146. Evrensel, Alper and Mehmet Emin Ceylan. "The Gut-Brain Axis: The Missing Link in Depression." *Clinical Psychopharmacology and Neuroscience.* December 2105. https://www.ncbi.nlm.nih.gov/pmc/articles/PMC4662178/
147. Gaynor, Mitchell M.D. "Diet and Depression" *Psychology Today October 25, 2014* https://www.psychologytoday.com/us/blog/your-genetic-destiny/201410/diet-and-depression
148. Valles-Colomer, Mireia, Gwen Falony, Youssef Darzi, *et al.* "The neuroactive potential of the human gut microbiota in quality of life and depression." *Nature Microbiology.* April 2019 https://www.nature.com/articles/s41564-018-0337-x.epdf
149. Naish, John. "Feeling low? It could be your antibiotics." IOL:Health & Wellness. June 7, 2016 https://www.iol.co.za/lifestyle/health/feeling-low-it-could-be-your-antibiotics-2031361
150. Handwerk, Brian. "Does Having a C-Section Alter Baby's First Microbiome?" Brian Handwerk. smithsonian.com February 1, 2016 https://www.smithsonianmag.com/science-nature/does-having-c-section-alter-babys-first-microbiome-180958002/#XAzhg6UCsj8xbHZx.99
151. Guaraldi, Federica and Guglielmo Salvatori. "Effect of Breast and Formula Feeding on Gut Microbiota Shaping in Newborns." *Frontiers in Cellular and Infection Microbiology* https://www.ncbi.nlm.nih.gov/pmc/articles/PMC3472256/

152. Lee, Stephanie. " In Treating Depression, Drugs Are Not Enough." Dr. Gabor Mate.com https://drgabormate.com/treating-depression-drugs-not-enough/

153. "Benzodiazepines and Opioids." National Institute on Drug Abuse. March 2018 https://www.drugabuse.gov/drugs-abuse/opioids/benzodiazepines-opioids

154. American Psychiatric Association. *Diagnostic and Statistical Manual of Mental Disorders.* Fourth Edition. Washington, DC: American Psychiatric Association, 2000. https://danya.com/dlc/bup/pdf/dependence_dsm.pdf

155. "Common Comorbidities with Substance Use Disorders." National Institute on Drug Abuse Advancing Addiction Science. https://www.drugabuse.gov/publications/research-reports/common-comorbidities-substance-use-disorders/part-1-connection-between-substance-use-disorders-mental-illness

156. Conway, Kevin P. PhD; Wilson Compton, MD, MPE; Frederick S. Stinson, PhD; and Bridget F. Grant, PhD. "Lifetime comorbidity of DSM-IV mood and anxiety disorders and specific drug use disorders: results from the National Epidemiologic Survey on Alcohol and Related Conditions." *Journal of Clinical Psychiatry.* February 2006. http://www.psychiatrist.com/JCP/article/Pages/2006/v67n02/v67n02 11.aspx

157. Brady, Kathleen T. M.D., Ph.D. "Comorbidity with Substance Abuse." *Medscape.* July 15, 2018 https://www.medscape.org/viewarticle/457178

158. "Benzodiazepines and Opioids." National Institute on Druge Abuse. March 2018. https://www.drugabuse.gov/drugs-abuse/opioids/benzodiazepines-opioids

159. Park, Tae Woo, Richard Saitz, Dara Gazoczy, Mark A. Ilgen and Amy S. B. Bohnert. "Benzodiazepine prescribing patterns and deaths from drug overdose among US veterans receiving opioid analgesics:

case-cohort study." *The British Medical Journal.* June 10, 2015. https://www.ncbi.nlm.nih.gov/pmc/articles/PMC4462713/

160. Vestal, Christine. " These Pills Could Be Next U.S. Drug Epidemic, Public Health Officials Say." Pew Trusts. July 18, 2018. https://www.pewtrusts.org/en/research-and-analysis/blogs/stateline/2018/07/18/these-pills-could-be-next-us-drug-epidemic-public-health-officials-say

161. "This Prescription Drug Is Implicated In Almost A Third Of All Opioid Overdose Deaths." *Huffington Post Wellness* March 15, 2017 https://www.huffingtonpost.com/entry/opioid-overdoses-combination-benzodiazepine_us_58c83e16e4b01c029d76f5ad

162. Lembke, Anna M.D. *Drug Dealer, M.D.* published in 2016 by Johns Hopkins University Press, 2016, Baltimore

163. "Prescription Opioid Data: Overdose Deaths Involving Prescription Opioids." Centers for Disease Control and Prevention https://www.cdc.gov/drugoverdose/data/prescribing.html

164. National Institute on Drug Abuse. "Overdose Death Rates." https://www.drugabuse.gov/related-topics/trends-statistics/overdose-death-rates

165. Siegel, Marc M.D. "The Opioid Contagion." Fox News. October 19, 2017. http://www.foxnews.com/opinion/2017/10/19/dr-marc-siegel-opioid-contagion.html

166. Leung, Pamela T.M., Erin M. Macdonald, M.Sc., Matthew B. Stanbrook, M.D., Ph.D., Irfan A. Dhalla, M.D., David N. Juurlink, M.D., Ph.D. "A 1980 Letter on the Risk of Opioid Addiction" *New England Journal of Medicine.* June 1, 2017 https://www.nejm.org/doi/full/10.1056/NEJMc1700150

167. Lurie, Julia. "A Brief, Blood-Boiling History of the Opioid Epidemic." *Mother Jones.* January/February 2017. https://www.motherjones.com/crime-justice/2017/12/a-brief-blood-boiling-history-of-the-opioid-epidemic/

168. Lurie, Julia. "A Brief, Blood-Boiling History of the Opioid Epidemic." *Mother Jones.* January/February 2017.

https://www.motherjones.com/crime-justice/2017/12/a-brief-blood-boiling-history-of-the-opioid-epidemic/

169. Perez-Pena, Richard. "Ohio Sues Drug Makers, Saying They Aided Opioid Epidemic." *The New York Times.* May 31, 2017 https://www.nytimes.com/2017/05/31/us/ohio-sues-pharmaceutical-drug-opioid-epidemic-mike-dewine.html

170. Centers for Disease Control and Prevention. "U.S. Opioid Prescribing Rate Maps." https://www.cdc.gov/drugoverdose/maps/rxrate-maps.html

171. Genetics Home Reference. "Opioid Addiction." National Institute Of Health. https://ghr.nlm.nih.gov/condition/opioid-addiction#statistics

172. National Institute on Drug Abuse. "Comorbidity: Substance Use Disorders and Other Mental Illnesses. Drug Facts. August 2018. https://d14rmgtrwzf5a.cloudfront.net/sites/default/files/drugfacts-comorbidity.pdf

173. Massing, Michael. "The Real Scandal in the Fight Against Opioids." *Politico Magazine.* July 21, 2018. https://www.politico.com/magazine/story/2018/07/21/opioids-treatment-politicians-media-219023

174. Andrews, Michelle. "Parents May Be Refused Details Of Adult Children's Medical Care." May 31 2016 Shots: Health News from NPR. https://www.npr.org/sections/health-shots/2016/05/31/479751997/parents-may-be-refused-details-of-adult-childrens-medical-care

175. "How HIPAA Prevents Seriously Mentally Ill from getting good care and what to do about." Mental Illness Policy Org. https://mentalillnesspolicy.org/wp-content/uploads/HIPAA_handcuffs.pdf

176. Gold, Jenny. "Privacy Law Frustrates Parents Of Mentally Ill Adult Children" Shots: Health News from NPR. June 4, 2014 https://www.npr.org/sections/health-shots/2014/06/04/318765929/privacy-law-frustrates-parents-of-mentally-ill-adult-children

177. Gold, Jenny. "Privacy Law Frustrates Parents Of Mentally Ill Adult Children" Shots: Health News from NPR. June 4, 2014 https://www.npr.org/sections/health-shots/2014/06/04/318765929/privacy-law-frustrates-parents-of-mentally-ill-adult-children

178. "H.R.2646 - Helping Families in Mental Health Crisis Act of 2016." Congress.gov https://www.congress.gov/bill/114th-congress/house-bill/2646

179. U.S. Department of Health and Human Services Office for Civil Rights "HIPAA Helps Caregiving Connections" https://www.hhs.gov/sites/default/files/hipaa-helps-stay-connected.pdf

180. "How HIPAA Prevents Seriously Mentally Ill from getting good care and what to do about." Mental Illness Policy Org. https://mentalillnesspolicy.org/wp-content/uploads/HIPAA_handcuffs.pdf

181. Gold, Jenny. "Parents Of Mentally Ill Adult Children Frustrated By Privacy Law." Kaiser Health News. June 5, 2014. https://khn.org/news/parents-of-mentally-ill-adult-children-frustrated-by-privacy-law/

182. Sederer, Lloyd I. M.D., Steven S. M.D. Sharfstein, MD. "Fixing the Troubled Mental Health System." *Psychology Today.* October 19, 2014. https://www.psychologytoday.com/us/blog/therapy-it-s-more-just-talk/201410/fixing-the-broken-mental-health-system

183. Greenberg, P.E., A.A. Fournier, T. Sisitsky, C. T. Pike and R.C. Kessler. "The economic burden of adults with major depressive disorder in the United States (2005 and 2010)." *Journal of Clinical Psychiatry.* February 2015 https://www.ncbi.nlm.nih.gov/pubmed/25742202

184. Daley, Dennis C. "Family and social aspects of substance use disorders and treatment." *Journal of Food and Drug Analysis.* December 2013. https://www.ncbi.nlm.nih.gov/pmc/articles/PMC4158844/

185. "Mental Health: A Report of the Surgeon General."
     https://profiles.nlm.nih.gov/ps/access/nnbbhy.pdf

Made in the USA
Monee, IL
16 September 2021

78233919R00115